This Side of Alcohol

Random thoughts
and candid words of pain, hope, humor, love ...
and all that is possible in sobriety-

Peggi Cooney

Leaning Rock Press
Gales Ferry, CT

Leaning Rock Press, LLC
Gales Ferry, CT 06335
leaningrockpress@gmail.com
www.leaningrockpress.com

978-1-950323-60-9, Hardcover
978-1-950323-61-6, Softcover
978-1-950323-62-3, eBook

Cover design by Kaitlyn Ash

Library of Congress Control Number: 2021914955

Publisher's Cataloging-In-Publication Data
(Prepared by The Donohue Group, Inc.)

Names: Cooney, Peggi, author.
Title: This side of alcohol : random thoughts and candid words of pain, hope, humor, love ... and all that is possible in sobriety / Peggi Cooney.
Description: Gales Ferry, CT : Leaning Rock Press, [2021] | Includes bibliographical references.
Identifiers: ISBN 9781950323609 (hardcover) | ISBN 9781950323616 (softcover) | ISBN 9781950323623 (ebook)
Subjects: LCSH: Cooney, Peggi--Diaries. | Recovering alcoholics--Biography. | Recovering alcoholics--Diaries. | Alcoholism--Psychological aspects. | LCGFT: Diaries. | Autobiographies.
Classification: LCC HV5293.C66 A3 2021 (print) | LCC HV5293.C66 (ebook) | DDC 362.292092--dc23

Printed in the United States of America

For my husband, Paul,
who chose to understand addiction over leaving.

For my children:
Matthew, Lindsay, and Brett

PRAISE FOR This Side of Alcohol

"What an inspiration! Peggi's story is one that resonates deeply with me and I appreciate her candor and forthrightness about a difficult topic. She's simultaneously encouraging and inspiring for anyone who finds herself in similar shoes. Taking control of life and going in a new direction is always a challenge, but Peggi has shared her brave story in a way that is engaging and relatable."
 – Keela Johnson, Forsyth Woman Magazine

"Peggi is the best kind of memoirist, one who is achingly honest, insightful and witty. The lessons in these pages will bring you to that special intersection of your heart and mind."
 – Kezia Calvert, The Sober Elephant Chronicles

"Peggi's raw no holds barred account of life in a bottle is an important contribution to a global conversation on alcohol and women."
 – Susan Christina, Founder of Hola Sober Magazine

"It wasn't until I read Peggi's story that I began to understand my own."
 – Jeff Graham, Getting BAC2ero

"Peggi's story is a life changer. I have seen it..a lot of it. She is no BS...completely devoted to the truth. A must read."
 – Michael McNamara, Founder of Post Traumatic Winning

"The Book is such a vivid, raw description of 'rock bottom reality' and the tricks that both alcohol and denial play on the mind. Peggi's powerful journey back to life makes us all believer that ANYTHING IS POSSIBLE!!"
 —Staci Danford, The Grateful Brain.

"Vulnerable, painful, hopeful and inspiring. In sharing her sobriety journey with us, Peggi lets us into her innermost thoughts and personal experiences as well as sharing the pointers she found along the way. This isn't just a 'how I did it' story but a guide to how you could do it too. In true Peggi style, she puts herself on the page so that others can can find a way out too."
 —Louise Atthey, author of Pearls of Wisdom

Chapter One

...And My Last Day One

"My family had my drinking problem."
—Jeff Graham

I think of July 11, 2019, as the final rock bottom that nearly cost me everything.

I was addicted to wine.

I still wake up to thoughts of that day. A day that was to be the finale. The finish. The closing act of my relationship with alcohol. My last day of playing Russian roulette with my family, my marriage, my career, and most of all, myself.

My husband, Paul, and I had just returned to the beautiful cabin in Lake Tahoe we rented for our annual family picnic at Sand Harbor. I purposely didn't drink at the reunion because I didn't want to do anything that would embarrass my family. So, I drank when I got back to the cabin. Quickly. And I had just spent eight hours in the sun, so the alcohol hit me like a brick.

A couple of hours later, my son Brett, daughter Lindsay, son-in-law Jason, and their two sets of twins (ages three and seven at the time) came home to find Paul screaming at me because I had been drinking. Again.

Brett, thinking he needed to defend me, went after Paul. Jason had to grab Brett to stop him. Lindsay and her children, my terrified grandchildren, stood there watching all of it. Paul left, with no intention of returning after 34 years of marriage. The rest of the night was a blur. I couldn't have hated myself any more than I did that night. I couldn't have been more broken.

The next morning, my quiet, reserved, more-mature-than-me daughter sat down across from me and said, "Mom, if you don't do something about your drinking, you cannot have the relationship you want with me, Jason and the kids." Her words broke my heart.

Painful words from a daughter who saw her mother drinking way too much at her best friend's wedding, passing out at her mother-in-law's home on Mother's Day, and being too drunk to babysit for her after another granddaughter's birthday party. All these events were followed by intense self-loathing and regret, yet apparently, none of them were rock bottom enough for me.

A daughter who, at two months pregnant with her first set of twins, left our house to go home because she didn't want her babies to feel the tension between Paul and me, who were once again having a heated argument that probably had something to do with my drinking.

A daughter who was totally onto me about my pre-party drinking. I had stopped drinking around her months before and instead stealthily—or so I thought—drank my wine before I would come over.

Now, I breathe and remind myself I am no longer that person. I am actually grateful to have had a tangible incident that ignited my resolve to stop drinking.

For good.

I'm not sure if Lindsay continues to see my drinking as a weakness, and that's okay. This is MY thing. I own it. My mother never had that chance. I thank God every day for my little girl, who in second grade was asked in a school project, "What is your favorite thing about your mom?" and answered, "I like my mom's neck." Really, Lindsay, the only thing you could come up with was my neck?

Although I will always credit my daughter's words that July day as the ones I needed to hear, words that literally saved my life, I also think about my son who stayed with me after Paul left. Brett watched over me to get me through those first couple of days when I was filled with complete self-hatred. This kid stayed with me while the others spent the day at the beach. (I was grateful they went to be with other family. The shame was almost unbearable.) Brett took me to lunch at a restaurant where I could barely keep from laying my aching head on the table. Just seeing and smelling his chili cheese fries came close to making me hurl.

I was conscious enough, however, to realize I had to do something as soon as possible that would make my family understand that I was serious about addressing my drinking. That same day, a Facebook advertisement popped up on my feed for Jenn Kautsch's Sober Sis 21 Day Reset program. I immediately signed up. The timing of this program appearing before me was no accident. It was a genuine gift from God.

That evening, while the others were still at the beach, I asked Brett to take me to an AA meeting. As I was walking into the meeting, I looked back at him in his car. He was crying.

I know he was scared.

I'll never forget how a man from AA witnessed this, walked over to my son, praised him for bringing me, and asked if there was anything he could do for him. He sat with Brett, and they talked for a few minutes. He even came out of the meeting and checked on Brett again. The people in the meeting gave me a Big Book that belonged to a long-time member who had passed away. The book was full of highlighted words and handwritten notes in the margins. These people had never met me before and will probably never see me again, yet they were exactly what I needed that night. There are so many kind and compassionate people in the world. You will find many of them in the rooms of AA.

Several years before this night, I started going to AA meetings in the small town near our cabin after one of the many times Paul left me because of my drinking. I'll never forget those people. They took me in when I was at one of the lowest points in my life. Little did I know, there would be an even lower point to come. I continued to attend meetings and I managed to stay sober for several months, but it didn't last. A couple months before I stopped for good, I ran into one of the women from the group at the grocery store and I had a bottle of wine in my cart. I heard myself telling her the wine wasn't for me.

Two years later (that's 731 days, for those of you who are counting, because I know I do), Brett still calls me almost every day. He does so not to check on me, but to check in with me. We have meaningful conversations about life, and I remember all of them.

Even though Brett never really thought I had a serious drinking problem, he is clearly no longer worried about me. I am present. I am his mother. All is as it should be.

> "Such is the strength of denial when it comes to drinking ... that a child talking to their parent may not even hit home" [1] —Talitha Cummins

Thank God I listened. My daughter now has a predictable mother upon whom she and her children can depend every single day; a daughter who usually shows her affection by texting the "thumbs up" emoji and acknowledges my sober milestones with hearts and the treasured words, "I am proud of you." I can feel the connection with her even though she has a harder time talking about it. She calls me now for no apparent reason, something she hadn't done in a while.

Before I stopped drinking, I spent hours on the internet searching to see if I really had a drinking problem—more times than not, with a glass of sauvignon blanc in my hand. And, of course, the internet makes it possible to find a source to support any opinion under the sun, no matter how outrageously unscientific it might be. Just the fact that I was looking on the internet to see how "bad" my drinking was should have been my first clue, right? Nope, because I could always find a reason for concluding that things weren't THAT bad, whatever "THAT" means.

I ignored that small voice inside that was telling me the truth the whole time; I refused to listen, because I just wasn't ready. Until I was. Now I listen to that voice every day and I can feel in my head, heart, and body that alcohol has lost its grip on me.

How did it happen? Well, I did something that was in stark contrast to my usual modus operandi when things went south, which was to retreat, wallow in self-loathing, hide in my house, and drink. This time I reached out and asked for help.

I cannot adequately describe the emotional pain I was in for the first three months of my sobriety. My marriage was falling apart. I was so full of guilt and shame that I was physically sick. And in the middle of all this, my brother Bob suffered a massive heart attack and almost died. He was in a coma for weeks and in the hospital for what seemed like forever.

Three things kept me going: my children, my grandchildren, and that voice I heard on my last day one, when I was literally down on my knees in the bedroom of the Lake Tahoe cabin—the voice that quietly, but clearly, said to me: "Peggi, you are done—and you are going to be okay."

I had to get uncomfortable, doing the things that I never would have seen myself doing before.

It was time to get busy. I totally immersed myself in everything sober by journaling every day, reading books, listening to podcasts, and then journaling some more. When the Sober Sis Reset program started, I had nineteen days of sobriety under my belt and poured myself (irony duly noted) into the daily lessons. The program also included being put into a group of about 25 women from all over the country. Called "Marco Polo," the group relies on communication among members through video-posting, in a walkie-talkie-like fashion. Bottom line, I don't think I could have gotten sober without the support of these women, with many of whom I have established extremely close friendships.

I know from my training in social work that it takes about 21 days to form a habit and about 90 days to make it stick. The more time I put in, the more confident I became that I could actually do this sober thing.

Here are some of the things I did in that first month: mani-pedis with my daughter and grandkids, along with almost daily visits; connected daily with my Marco Polo group; made plans to attend the Sober Sis retreat in Fort Worth; and made lunch plans with new sober sisters. I drove to San Francisco with a sober sister to meet another to celebrate our successful 21-day reset.

At about 90 days AF (alcohol free; this acronym took some time to get used to), I started posting observations about my new alcohol-free lifestyle on social media. I wrote about the incredibly dumb-ass things I had routinely done to hide my drinking, things no normal drinker would ever consider doing (or would have to do). I also posted observations on how my life was improving as my AF days added up. I had no plans about how long I would continue posting. I was living day-to-day, and the posts just made me feel connected and accountable to my recovery community. Although my family was supportive of my sobriety, they really weren't into talking about it. I noticed how my writing was resonating with so many others. So, I kept posting. Every day. This book, one I never knew I would write, is the result of all those posts.

An interesting side effect of becoming sober minded was the opening of my eyes to the incredible pressure there is to drink in the US. I asked myself: When did it become okay to drink alcohol at a six-year-old's birthday party? When did it become a thing to take your children trick-or-treating with your wine glass in hand so that you can get your treat, too, at nearly every house in the neighborhood? When did grocery stores feel the need to open full-service bars in the middle of the food aisles? The tipping point for me was taking my three- and seven-year-old twin grandchildren to Disney on Ice, and having a dad spill a 40-ounce beer down my back. Seriously, beer, wine, and hard liquor offerings at a Disney matinee? And just recently, someone shared that her local zoo offers canned wine, hard seltzer, and a margarita machine. We can't even visit the zoo without booze?

Anyway …

I continued working on my sobriety by reading every "quit lit" book I could get my hands on, by listening to hundreds of hours of podcasts, and by enrolling in alcohol recovery-related programs such as Staci Danford's Gratitude Boost, Annie Grace's 100 Day Challenge, Laura McKowen's We Are the Luckiest: Sobriety in Full Color and Jenn Kautsch's Sober Sis Alcohol-Free Living. I'd put 150% into drinking; I got sober the same way.

At about one year into my sobriety, I felt the transformation from being an observer to being the director of my life. I was no longer getting sober for others. No more faking it until I made it. Sober became who I was. The work I had immersed myself in was paying off, and I literally felt reborn.

Breaking up with alcohol was like losing a relationship. We develop an emotional attachment to alcohol, just like with do with people and with our pets. I didn't know how to live without it. I also knew that if I didn't change my life, it would kill me. My breakup with booze was sad and hard and full of grief. I knew I was done drinking, yet it often felt devastating. I had to move through the stages of grief that made sense only to me. Sobriety forces you to look at your life, and I had never done that before—at least, not in any meaningful way. I had to learn to love myself, and that wasn't a simple thing to do.

The road to self-love and self-acceptance isn't a straight one. Life gets "lifey" (thank you, Meegan Baxter), but it also gets better, so much better.

The work continues. There is always that next meeting, that book, that post, that podcast, that program or course, that conversation, that lifting of another person who is struggling with their own relationship with alcohol.

There is the honesty that comes with sobriety. I don't know how to be anything but transparent in my storytelling. The truth has literally set me free.

My friend Louise said, "I don't want to get to the end. I just want to go on. I used to live in quicksand. Now I am slipping on solid rock. I am ready to learn the things I am supposed to learn when I am presented with them. Joy is in the journey."

Yes, Louise, it is.

Chapter Two

Letters to Bill and Margaret

"Not your fault, not mine, just is."
—Katherine Fabrizio

"We are all wounded deer in life's forest
trying to find our way."
—Lucy Tosti

I grew up in what I would consider a middle-class home in San Leandro, California, a once small, now large San Francisco Bay Area suburb. My dad, Bill, was an automobile service manager, and my mother, Margaret, was a homemaker with occasional part-time jobs. I have two half-brothers, Jerry and Jim, eight and ten years older than me. Their father died from a brain tumor at 29. Ten years later, my mother married Bill. Soon after, I was born, weighing seven pounds, 14 ounces. My mom chose to call me Peggi, which is supposedly a nickname for "Margaret." I will never understand the connection. My grandmother Julie called my mom "Peggi" when she was good and "Margaret" when she wasn't. Ten years after I was born, my mother gave birth to my brother Bob. Jim postponed his wedding so that Mom wouldn't be walking down the aisle in a maternity dress.

A quick math calculation will therefore reveal that there is a 20-year age difference between my oldest and youngest siblings. This naturally makes for interesting "family tree" questions, more so because Bob (aka youngest brother) went to live with Jim (aka oldest brother) when he was nine years old, thus begging the question from my kids, "Is Bob our uncle or our cousin?" Yes. These interesting dynamics came together when my son Brett was asked in the third grade, "What do you want to be when you grow up?" and he replied, "I want to grow up, get married, get divorced and be an uncle." This was, of course, followed by a phone call from his concerned teacher. I had to explain to Brett that getting married and divorced weren't prerequisites for uncle status.

My parents' relationship was always a rocky one. There was a constant stream of intimate partner violence in our home. There was a lot of screaming, throwing, leaving and long periods of sometimes almost unbearable silence. I'm pretty sure that infidelity found its way in there somewhere, too. (Case in point: the lipstick on my father's forehead that wasn't my mother's.) I realize, now, that alcohol fueled all of it.

One of my earliest memories was from when I was about three and my mom decided to trim my bangs which, thereafter, always sparked controversy between my parents. Mom had a difficult time making my bangs even and she would alternately trim one side, then the other, until all that I had left was about a quarter of an inch of hair running along the top of my forehead. I have pictures to prove it. Hair got in my eyes and made me cry. Then Dad would come home and yell at Mom, "Shit, Margaret, what did you do to her?" Which would make me cry more. (I never attempted to cut or trim any of my kids' hair.)

And yet, there was love, too. They seemed to love each other as much as they fought. There were lots of family trips and vacations, boating, barbequing and other adventures. My parents were very social and had lots of friends. At times, they were openly affectionate with each other. At other times, they were mortal enemies. If my dad criticized my mom, her modus operandi was to throw anything she had in her hand at his head. If he made a comment that his soft-boiled egg wasn't soft enough, she would likely throw it at him. Or if the blueberry muffins were undercooked? Watch out! We often had to duck to avoid being hit by a flying muffin tray. That combination made for a real eggshell life for me and my siblings. Both of my older brothers left home as soon as they could. Our little brother was born when my mom was 43 and both Jim and Jerry were already out on their own.

My parents divorced about nine years later. Mom's rheumatoid arthritis was progressing fast, and by the time we moved to be closer to her sister, she could no longer work and had to go on welfare. That completely humiliated her. Dad got remarried six months later—to a woman who looked like Mom, only she wasn't sick.

Moving to a new school in the middle of my junior year of high school was quite traumatic. My new history teacher introduced me to a guy who was about to go on his Mormon mission. The poor guy's plans changed when I got pregnant. I finished high school in Provo, Utah, where our daughter, Shi, was born. I was three weeks short of turning 18. Finances forced us to move back to California and shortly thereafter, our daughter died. She strangled at my brother's house while my ex-sister-in-law was babysitting her. My heart was broken. Our marriage didn't survive the loss. Neither did my brother's.

I lost my identity. I was no longer a mother. I was still in my teens, yet I was hardly a teenager. My parents died before my 20th birthday. I spent the next several years going to school, working and traveling, doing a lot of growing and screwing up. I remarried at 27, to my kids' dad, Sonny. We met at Cattlemen's Steak House, where we both worked as servers. A great guy, he did nothing to contribute to the demise of our seven-year marriage. I think I was attracted to Sonny because he was so hard working and stable. He was still living at home when we met, and I was so impressed with how dedicated his parents were to each other and to their five children. I had no idea what a healthy marriage looked like. Sonny and I did a good job of co-parenting after our divorce. His parents, Walt and Ida, were the best and the only grandparents my children knew. They were everything to our kids. And after they forgave me for leaving the marriage, they treated me with nothing but love and kindness.

Two years later, I married for the third time. Blended families are inherently challenging. When Paul and I got married 35 years ago, G and L were nine and 12; my kids were three, five and six. They were all beautiful humans who were thrown together in a family of which none of them asked to be a part. At 34, I had no clue how to be a stepmother. Loaded with great intentions, I never once tried to take the place of their mother or to push them into liking me. I understood what it was like to be in a stepfamily because I had lived in one myself.

I didn't know where I fit in (who did?) and I was often nervous and moody around my stepdaughters. "Crazy" was a word that G used several times to describe me to others. Paul and I argued a lot, mostly about the kids. My defense mechanisms kicked in when he tried to discipline mine; I would accuse him of favoring his. (Of course he did.) I made so many mistakes and constantly told myself I wasn't trying hard enough. I'm quite sure this was the foundation of my self-doubt, which would rear its ugly head many times going forward.

Something that sticks out to me is how unconditionally kind G and L were to my kids. Their kindness has continued into adulthood.

It certainly wasn't all negative. We built memories and went on trips—to Crater Lake, Disneyland, the family cabin in Lake Tahoe. Our aerobics/dance/art/theater studio became a family thing. We created many of our own traditions. I spent hours sewing everyone Christmas stockings.

I loved watching all the kids grow up and grow out of the house to create families of their own, none of which included divorce, thank God. And I'll always be beyond grateful for how G and L have let me be a real grandmother to their five amazing children.

Being a stepmother can be a lonely role. Paul treated me differently in front of G and L. I began to feel resentful. During the last decade, I drank more to reduce the anxiety I felt when I was around them, and as you can imagine, there were some not-so-proud stepmother moments courtesy of alcohol. My behavior made them more guarded around me; I became withdrawn around them. My drinking only worked to reinforce the way they felt about me.

Drinking didn't become a problem for me until I was in my fifties. Until then, I drank socially, and I really thought little about it. Looking back, it's clear that when I drank, I rarely stopped at one, and often wouldn't stop until I reached the level of what one would consider "binge drinking." It took me awhile, but I now recognize I had re-created the very relationship with alcohol my parents had.

Alcohol certainly played a part in why I had to live most of my adult life without my parents.

***

Dear Dad:

You walked off that golf course and a widow maker took you from us at age 47. I was 19, and the world as I knew it, ceased to exist. I was still reeling from losing your nine-month-old granddaughter to an accident that would fracture our family for years. You were my only solace, my only comfort. Little did I know I was about to lose Mom, too. You died from the perfect storm: high blood pressure, smoking, and I'm pretty sure alcohol played a role.

I'm not sure why I was never angry with you for leaving me like I was with Mom.

I think it might have been your complete love for life. You loved everyone and everyone loved you back. There were hundreds of people at your funeral. Remember when you went out for antifreeze for the car and you came home with a new car because it came with antifreeze? Mom was so pissed.

I remember you waterskiing by taking off from the beach, donning your favorite straw hat, holding your cigarette (so very sophisticated at the time), waterskiing around the lake, getting dropped off, kicking off your skis as you walked up on the beach, and stamping out your cigarette in the sand like it was nothing. You were absolutely the coolest person I knew.

I loved it when you let me be your golf caddy. Until that one day I flipped the cart upside-down.

I loved being the just-one-onion-two-olive garnish maker for your martinis.

I loved how you took care of Mom after the divorce by mowing her lawn and just checking in on her.

I hated you both for getting divorced in the middle of my junior year of high school and having to move to a new town with complete strangers. At 17, I got back at you by making you grandparents for the fifth time.

I inherited your sense of humor, your love of life, your impulsiveness, your sense of adventure and your love of alcohol. I almost followed in your footsteps, Dad, but that will not be my legacy now. My children will never have to write a letter like this. I miss you, Dad. Every day. I get to see you often, though, because your grandson Brett is your clone in every way possible. He is charming and impulsive. Hilarious. Compassionate. And, at almost eight years of age, your great-granddaughter Teagan is learning to play golf. I told her all about you.

***

Dear Mom:

The official cause was rheumatoid arthritis and pneumonia, but we both know that alcohol was also responsible for you leaving this earth at age 51. I was 19. Bob, Jerry, and Jim were nine, 27 and 29. All these years, 49 of them without you now, I have been so angry with you for all the things you missed: my college graduations, my careers, your grandkids and great-grandkids, my successes, and my fuckups. I inherited your creativity, your love of reading, and your struggle with alcohol. Oh, and I suck at cooking, just like you. (Remember how our dog, Sam, was so skinny?)

I was walking this morning, and I was thinking about how much you would have loved reading *This Naked Mind, We Are the Luckiest, The Sober Diaries,* and *Drinking: A Love Story.* You would have loved Sober Sis and The Luckiest Club. I was thinking how those books and these amazing communities might have changed the trajectory of your life as they have mine. Mom, I know you would have loved the science behind it all. For me, it hasn't only given me sobriety, but the grace to forgive you because now I know it wasn't your fault. I'm no longer pissed off every time I think of you.

I never appreciated your growing up during the Depression with five siblings and how hard that must have been. I didn't have the compassion you deserved for becoming a widow with two young boys when you were just 29 years old. Or the years you suffered with debilitating and painful arthritis. I do now.

This past Christmas, I put out some of your decorations and looked at them with a new appreciation for, and a renewed connection to, you.

I am finally at peace. I hope you are, too. I love you, Mom. Someday I will tell you all about it.

Chapter Three

Unfiltered
(The first 90 days)

"New beginnings are often disguised as painful endings."
—Lau Tzu

I had been outsourcing my feelings to alcohol for years—sadness, happiness, anxiety, all of it. I drank to forget; I drank to cope, albeit temporarily with all the stresses and conflicts in my life. Yet, no matter how much I drank, all those negative emotions would come back in spades. So many of us know that feeling of waking up the next day in a pool of shame, scanning our phones, clothes, or kitchen for evidence of the damage and self-destruction. On my last day one, when I was at the lowest place in my life, I was disconnected from everyone. I was disconnected from myself.

Those first 90 days were rough. When I stopped drinking, I was flooded with negative emotions that I had shoved down with wine for years. I didn't know how to allow myself to experience them. They washed over me like a tsunami. I constantly felt like I had the flu. I had no energy.

The following words are some of my raw and unedited journal entries in the first 90 days of my sobriety. Cliff Notes summary: I was a total mess. I pulled it together for teaching, but that's about all I could do. Half-way through this first three months, my brother almost died. For weeks, I felt like I was just sitting in the hurt.

15

Themes of guilt and shame, anxiety and pain, ran deep. I couldn't see the "New Life Ahead" sign.

Yet, I didn't pick up that glass.

Day 2

Brett just dropped me off at the condo. On the ride home, he told me I should probably never drink around Lindsay again. I don't think I will drink around ANYONE again. It was all I could do to hold back the tears. Paul is gone. His closet is practically empty. I can't help but feel somewhat relieved that he isn't here because the thought of facing him seems even worse. Every one of my nerves is on fire. I have been crying my face off. I posted a video on Marco. I don't know what to do next.

Day 3

I have become someone I don't recognize.

Day 5

My emotions are all over the place. Last weekend saved my life and at the same time, I am so fucking pissed off. At everything and everyone. I haven't heard from Paul. Lindsay and Brett are checking up on me every day. It's painful that they think they have to do that, and yet, it's comforting somehow. I am scared out of my mind and yet somehow relieved that I can finally stop lying about this part of my life.

I am reading the book The Happier Hour, by Rebecca Weller. So much of her story resonates with mine. I am still trying to sort out how the hell I got to this place.

> "This was no way to live; constantly in fear of messing everything up. Why on earth was I self-sabotaging, anyway? I was THIS close to living my dream life, with a new career I was so passionate about and the-love-of-my-life by my side. Was I really choosing wine over wellness? Vodka over vitality? Tequila over tranquility? I

cried. The grief was all-encompassing and unrelenting. I sobbed, heart breaking tears of sadness for getting myself stuck in this mess." [2]

I thought to myself, Rebecca had a partner who loved her through her journey to sobriety. Her addiction was way worse than mine. (Such ridiculous things we tell ourselves—addiction is addiction.) Paul has put me down, called me names, stopped talking to me, left me, refused to let me come home. I feel flawed, like there is something so innately wrong with me. Like I have this irredeemable character defect. I'm wondering if Paul and I can even find our way to the other side of all of this. I'm not sure I even want to.

Day 7

I am currently reading Clare Pooley's The Sober Diaries. Reading about others who-were-where-I-am-now is somehow comforting. It makes me feel less lonely, like I'm not the only one on the entire planet going through this. Pooley's thoughts could be my thoughts:

> "Right now, I really need some friends. I need someone to hold my hand and tell me I can do this. I need someone to tell me what to expect. I need someone to tell me it's going to be okay in the end." [3]

Clare's husband, John, loved her through sobriety. I don't think Paul has the capacity or the desire to do that.

Day 10

I read that at ten days, all the alcohol has left my body. I also know I have been here many times before. Maybe this drinking thing isn't all my fault. Annie Grace offers another explanation, other than being weak, for allowing alcohol to take over my life:

> "Who is to blame? It seems society would have you believe it is you, the drinker. You probably believe that

your inability to control drinking—unlike 'regular drinkers' who 'can take it or leave it'—is because of a flaw you possess, and they don't. What if that's not true?" [4]

Reading her words makes me feel lighter today.

Day 11

I am a hot mess. I know the alcohol is completely out of my system and yet I'm terrified. I feel physically sick. I am miserable. I continue to cry my face off. I go to bed at 6:00 pm. Paul is still gone. I'm not sure if I want him to come back, but I don't want my drinking to be the reason he left.

Day 12

I am journaling and reading quit lit books like a complete madwoman. I appreciate the science behind alcohol addiction. I feel myself breathing more. I feel the fog lifting. I found Jason Vale's very frank words in *Kick the Drink* such a powerful argument for getting and staying sober:

> "If you pass out on alcohol, it means that your body cannot keep you alive and awake at the same time as it needs all of its resources to deal with the poison in the bloodstream ... you are effectively in a coma...
>
> The real questions should be, 'I can have a drink, but what on earth would be the point? What would it do for me?' The answer will be crystal clear—nothing...
>
> Oh, sorry, apart from the headaches, the hangovers, the lethargy, the bad breath, the beer gut, the arguments, the violence, being overemotional, regretting things you've done but can't remember doing, getting things out of proportion, putting off things all the time, the stress, the over-drafts, the taxis, the guilt, the lies, the deceit, the brewers droop, the mood swings, the breakdown of the immune system, the lack of resistances to all kinds of diseases, the destruction of brain cells, not to mention excess weight ..." [5]

Just, wow. I was slowly killing myself with alcohol.

Day 13

Paul came home for a couple days. It's excruciating having him here because he is so angry. I have been hiding in my room, keeping myself busy and trying to stay out of his way. I'm burying myself in reading, listening to podcasts, and journaling. I go to bed early to avoid him and to keep from getting too sad. The 21-day reset doesn't start for three more days. My only supports right now are my kids and my Marco group.

Paul just accused me of playing games. I don't even know what he means by that. I'm not sure where all this is going. The tension in this house is almost unbearable. Why is he even here?

I wrote a letter to my adult stepdaughters. Paul is angry I sent it to them without showing it to him first. I had no problem letting him read it. Why is he so upset I sent it? Makes me wonder what he told them. They weren't even there when this last incident happened.

L and G:

I am not sure where to begin and I don't feel confident enough to talk to you in person yet. I have so much to say, and I want to put down my words, go over them again, so that I can be sure they convey my most heartfelt intentions and feelings.

Since the picnic, I have attacked my drinking issues as if I am doing a full-scale research project. I have immersed myself in sober literature. I read six books, listened to hours of podcasts, I write daily in my journal and joined Sober Sis, which is an international women's group whose goal is to support women who want to live a sober-minded lifestyle. It was created by Jenn Kautsch, is based in Fort Worth, Texas and has several components: A 21-Day Reset where you commit to not drinking along with daily emails/activities, Zoom calls, Facebook, Marco Polo videos with a group of about 25 women, podcasts and other activities. I am seriously excited about what I am learning. I would love for you to go online to see what Sober Sis is about. Jenn's advertising kept popping up on my Facebook page, and I had seriously been contemplating about joining for several months, but when Friday happened, it was the first thing I did on Saturday morning. Brett also took me to an AA meeting on Saturday night.

I am registered and have my airfare for the Sober Sis retreat in Fort Worth on October 18–20.

During the past 14 days, I have learned what alcohol does to a woman's mind, body, and soul. It is literally poison, more addictive and harmful than heroin, crack, crystal meth and cocaine. I have fallen in love with the brain science behind alcohol addiction. I teach about brain science and it fits in with everything I know. Alcohol doesn't satisfy the desire to drink alcohol. I know for sure, that being anxious about attending certain social events influenced my drinking. And I know now that alcohol creates more anxiety, it doesn't take it away. I have learned that alcohol affects every organ of your body, no matter how little or how much you drink. Alcohol can weaken the heart muscle, affect our electrical system, can cause blood clots, increase strokes by 39%, stretch blood vessels, increase blood pressure, affect liver function, immune system and can cause cancer.

It obviously can influence relationships, and right now, I have pretty much flipped my family on its head.

I don't even know if the relationship between Brett and Paul can ever be repaired. I hope time and the fact that I have committed to sobriety might help. I know (from your dad) that both of you think I should go into some structured facility to get help and that you have huge doubts I can stay sober. I can truly say I am not physically addicted to alcohol. I have had nothing to drink since July 12, and I do not crave it at all. As you know, alcohol has not always been an issue for me and really started in my 50s for a lot of reasons.

I talked to my doctor about what I am doing. She is so supportive. I told Lindsay and Brett as well. I still need to talk to Matt.

I know I have made a mess of things, but I have so much hope. I want to earn your trust again, not with my words, but with my actions. I am learning the tools I need to stay alcohol free, especially in social situations. I exercise daily. I am constantly reaching out to my support system in Sober Sis.

Paul is reading two of the "quit lit" books and we are having some meaningful conversations. He is learning that the shaming and blaming he did to try to get me to stop drinking only made things worse and is not an effective way to support a partner.

I am committed to this journey, no matter what happens. I want things to work out with you, my kids, and my marriage, but I am doing this for me, first. I have a dream job; I LOVE my work and I never want to jeopardize that. And I can actually be a better instructor because I will no longer take part in the hypocrisy of teaching social workers how to work with families affected by addiction.

I will never have another hangover, have to piece together horrifying gaps in my memory, apologize for my behavior. Like Jenn says, "No one has ever woken up feeling like they should have had a drink the night before."

I love you both. I am truly sorry for the pain I have caused.

Love, Peg

Day 14

Brett called today. He was justifiably angry because I put him in a position where, by feeling the need to go after Paul, he could have been arrested. I'm glad he could vent like that. It's true. It's not the first time I have put my sons in a situation where they felt the need to defend me. I did the same thing to Matt at a wedding we attended a few years ago. Another alcohol-fueled event that ended with Paul and me fighting because I lost my wallet.

Brett said that he would always support and love me, but that he is done with his stepfather. He wanted me to know that he will not be attending Christmas or any other holiday where Paul might be. I just listened and told him I understood. I do.

Day 16

I can't help but think the reunion weekend saved my life. I was not headed in a good direction.

Day 17

I decided to practice some self-care in the hot tub. Without wine, I felt every bubble. I felt my body relax for the first time in over two weeks. I took in the view like I was looking at it for the first time— the blue Mt. Lassen skies and the swaying leaves of the aspen trees that seem to be communicating with each other in their own secret and spiritual language. Everything seemed amplified, brighter. The flowers Paul planted are all in bloom in shades of pink, purple, yellow and white. The quail mothers and their babies were out in full force while the males held sentry on top of the boulders. Today has been a good day.

Day 20

Still haven't heard from L and G. It's been a week. I can totally understand why they don't believe that I am serious about getting sober this time. What I can't understand is getting no response at all, not one I-don't-believe-you or we-need-more-time-to-forgive-you. Nothing. After 33 years of being a family. Their support is non-existent. There must be something else going on.

Day 21

I dreamed I drank a screwdriver last night! The dream seemed so incredibly real. I hate orange juice (notice I didn't say I hate vodka). In the dream, I was looking at Paul, who was watching me in disgust. I cannot tell you how relieved I was when I woke up and realized it was just a dream. That really shook me up.

It's common for people to have dreams about drinking in early recovery. It turns out that those who wake up sad or disappointed that the dream wasn't real tend to be more prone to relapse. Those who wake up relieved tend to become more motivated to remain alcohol free. It's also thought that dreams may have a compensatory effect, allowing a person to deal with urges and cravings in a safe way (S.Y. Choy).

There is research that supports that the addicted brain is trying to reset itself. Drinking interferes with normal dream activity. You dream more when you stop drinking because you experience more REM sleep where dreams occur.

Day 22

I want to start a program like Sober Sis for our child welfare parents.

Day 23

I feel like I lost Brett. We had such a close relationship; now our conversations have boundaries—things we can't talk about. I'm grieving over this. And will Lindsay talk to me about any of this? She shuts down so easily. And I need to talk to Matt.

Day 24

Thank God for this summer slowdown in my teaching schedule. I can barely keep it together.

Day 25

I don't know if my marriage will survive this. Paul thinks I want this to be easy. He has come back home, but it feels more like a punishment than a reconciliation. I didn't ask him to come back home. He is calling me "selfish" with "a weak character." He accused me of "ripping this family apart at the seams."

He has agreed to read William Porter's book, *Alcohol Explained*. Maybe that will help. Shit, I get his anger and yet I'm resentful because some of my drinking was my way of coping with our relationship. Have I re-created my parents' relationship with Paul?

I am not drinking. I am not drinking. I am not drinking.

Day 26

I don't expect anyone to believe this at 26 days sober, but I'm certain I will never pick up another drink again. No matter what happens. I know I have said this before, but I can FEEL that this time is different. I can't explain it. I just KNOW.

Day 27

My psychologist is so supportive and agrees with all I am doing to maintain my sobriety. I gave her a copy of the letter I wrote to my stepdaughters. She encouraged me to give it time.

Day 28

I find myself studying how to be sober like I'm studying for another master's degree. I'm obsessed.

Day 30

I find myself not wanting to share any of my sobriety journey with Paul. Maybe because he shamed me in the past and I don't want to give him any more ammunition. He is reading books about addiction and supporting me on some levels, yet his past words still sting—alcoholic, mental, crazy, selfish. I disgust him. It's never been how he might help me, only that I embarrassed and humiliated him. I just don't like him at all right now. I want to shut him out. I know he is feeling it, too. I hope that as the days add up, I'll change my attitude and have compassion for what I have put him through. We have been married 33 years ...

Day 32

Paul and I went out for a Cold Stone ice cream tonight. We are so uncomfortable and awkward together. I don't even like ice cream.

Day 35

How do Paul and I manage the outrageously oversized elephant in the room? What did he say to his 40-something daughters that made them want nothing to do with me? What did he tell them that made them so angry? He won't tell me. I didn't drink at the family picnic, and they didn't see me THAT night. I don't even know what I am dealing with. The unknowing feels so hopeless and isolating.

I felt somewhat better after I talked to my Marco sisters. I was in so much pain when I shared what was going on, even Jenn from Sober Sis sent me a message.

Yet even this broken heart will not make me pick up that glass. I don't have to do anything other than not drink today.

Day 37

How many times did I convince Paul I was okay and that "this time" I had my drinking under control? I quit so many times, many of those for substantial periods, yet each time I went back, my drinking continued to escalate until I was nothing more than a human who lies. Will I ever get past this shame?

Day 38

Paul was talking on the phone to his daughter yesterday and I overheard him use the term "alcoholic" in reference to me. Ugh. I have no issue with people who choose to call themselves by that term. For me, it is a lifetime label that is shaming and judgmental. I am a person who happened to have a drinking problem. And now I don't.

Day 42

I am so furious right now that I am literally shaking. I feel completely betrayed. Disrespected. I just found out that Paul shared extremely personal details about our marriage with his daughters that he had absolutely no right to do. WTF? He says he regrets doing it, but he explained that at the time he did this, he was hurt and angry and had decided to end our marriage. Now it makes sense why they ignored my letter and attempts to make amends and why G never acknowledged the five doll outfits that I designed, created, and sent for her blanket business. Paul watched me doing it. Why didn't he stop me? I didn't know he had talked to her. No wonder G thought I was trying to manipulate her. Not true. Not true at all.

I take full responsibility for my drinking. I put Paul through hell the last ten years, but his sharing only one side of some very intimate details in our relationship was an extremely bonehead thing for him to do. G and L aren't going to forget the things he said to them. Our marriage feels like it's in big trouble.

Day 44

Paul mentioned that G and L think I need to go into rehab. During this conversation, Paul referred to me as an alcoholic. Again. I need to take a breath, maybe explain to him why being called an alcoholic is so shaming to me. And I need to let it go about G and L. I cannot make them like me, and my sobriety does not and cannot depend on their approval. I realize I have been seeking their approval our whole marriage. Lindsay pointed out to me that my drinking became a self-fulfilling prophecy.

I have spent years trying to fit in as a stepmother. Going forward, I will accept the relationship for what it is, not the fantasy I imagined it to be. There is a certain feeling of freedom with that kind of thinking. No expectations. I am so grateful for the role I have been able to play as a grandmother. That is what I will focus on.

Day 46

When my drinking became a problem, it wasn't about how Paul could help me; it was about how I embarrassed and/or humiliated him. I needed to decide on my own what was the next right thing. Threats and name calling seemed to make me dig in my heels and drink at him. Would I feel the same way if the roles were reversed? Possibly. I would like to think I would have approached it differently.

Day 47

Just got to the cabin. I saw that Paul threw out all the liquor in the house. At first, I was so hurt and filled (once again) with guilt and shame that he felt the need to do that. It was a reminder of the broken trust my drinking created. My first instinct was to pick up the phone and scream at him. I. DON'T. DRINK. ANY. MORE! I took a breath. After what I put him through, maybe it was cathartic for him. Or maybe he thought he was doing me a favor.

He really cannot know what is in my heart, and what is in my heart is that I have been done with drinking forever for 47 days.

Day 49

Paul said he gave G a copy of *This Naked Mind*. That was a very cool move.

.

Day 54

Yesterday, my brother Bob suffered a massive heart attack. I am sitting with him and his wife, Monica, at Mercy General in Sacramento waiting for the surgeon to arrive at any minute, and when he gets here, Bob will go straight into surgery. Please God, don't take my brother. Not for me (that's kind of a lie), but for his teenage sons, Luke and Jake.

After almost 12 grueling hours, Dr. S came out to tell us that Bob survived but there are no guarantees.

Even this early in sobriety, I have no desire to pick up a drink. I want to be here when Bob wakes up.

Day 57

My brother may not be able to hear me, but I know he knows I am here even if he can't respond. It's been three days and Bob hasn't woken up yet. That didn't keep me from talking to him whenever I could go in. One of the ICU nurses walked in while I was talking to my brother and said to me, "You know that it's useless to talk to him because he can't hear you." I broke into tears and eeked out, "He may not be able to hear me, but he can FEEL I am here even if he can't respond!"

Day 60

Dr S said ICU staff will push Bob hard today. They are worried about his lungs, which he described as being full of lots of green yucky stuff. (Is that a medical term?) The ICU will start giving him antibiotics and plan to ease him out of the coma and maybe by the end of the week, they can take him off the ventilator.

Day 65

Bob is improving ever so slowly. Understandably, there is a tension between me and my siblings. We are all just exhausted because we have been practically living at the hospital. And we are all scared. Yet now isn't the time, brother Jim, to bring up how you think your stepfather, my father, was an asshole. Geez, let it go!

Day 71

I texted Lindsay that I'm at 71 days alcohol free. She texted back that she is proud of me.

Later, Paul told me he was going to have a talk with his daughters. I suggested that might make things worse, that giving them time might be a better strategy. He disagreed, accusing me of trying to make him choose between his daughters and me, followed by, maybe he doesn't want to stay married. Ugh.

Day 75

My mental gymnastics:
I cannot drink anymore.
For the rest of my life.
Then who am I?
I won't ever have fun again.
I hate mocktails! They seem completely stupid to me.
I can order a club soda with a splash of cranberry or pomegranate with a squeeze of lime.
That will get old fast.
How boring.
Maybe no one will notice I am not drinking.
I hate big groups.
I don't want the focus on me.

If people see I am not drinking they will think I have a problem.
Fuck it.
Those are the people who don't like me anyway.
Then why do I feel like I must "prove" my sobriety to people that don't matter?
Fuck them.
Ugh. This is all so exhausting.

Day 85

Bob is being transferred to the rehab unit, his last stop before being able to go home. He is complaining about all the occupational and physical therapy he has to do every day. Hearing my brother bitch again is music to my ears.

Day 89

Now that Bob is out of the woods, I'll be leaving on a jet plane to Dallas/Fort Worth in a little over a week to attend the Sober Sis retreat. This will be my first alcohol-free event, I think, in almost ever. While I'm there, I will hit my 100-day milestone. I'll meet Jenn, and a few of my Marco sisters. I'm nervous and excited.

Day 90

Not one word from G & L. Who completely ignores a letter like I sent? Who does that? No "I got your letter, but I am so mad at you right now, I am not ready to talk." Not one "I am not ready to forgive you yet." Nothing. Nada.

Chapter Four

Early Observations
(Three to six months)

"The world's favorite drink is a drug."
—Clare Pooley

During the next three months, I experienced mood swings that rivaled Sybil's. There were days when it all felt so unbearably heavy and unending. I found myself exhausted from the constant chatter in my head—those thoughts, ideas, and dreams that, in the past, I only knew how to quiet with wine. My education in social work told me that this Jekyll-and-Hyde behavior was my brain and body adjusting to life without alcohol. This knowledge was of little comfort when I was welling up with tears or feeling intensely angry for no apparent reason. The phrase that I heard over and over in early sobriety—"you just have to feel the feels"—made me angry and often felt condescending. I was grieving an emotional attachment that I thought had served me well over the past decade. Until it didn't.

I spent so much time alternating between feelings of anger, shame or loneliness, and joy. One minute I would be filled with self-loathing and in the next, I would find myself on the proverbial "pink cloud," a term used to describe the euphoric feeling of being free from alcohol in early sobriety.

Slowly, I began the gradual climb to introspection, documented by journaling. My writing became a distraction from those all-over-the-place emotions coming out from a brain trying to regulate itself after being abused for a decade. Some days, all I could do was write in my journal, cross out the day with a big "X" in my planner, and go to bed. Like Elizabeth Kubler-Ross's theory of the five stages of grief, nothing was linear about my process or my journey on the emotional rollercoaster that is sobriety.

So, here it goes—my random journal writings and posts on getting and staying sober beginning on day 91. The entries run the gamut of emotions from sad to happy, scared to brave, alone to connected, resentful to grateful. It's all there; I don't think I left much out.

***

Today, at my big, beautiful grocery store with at least 15 checkout stands, this thought came to me; I will no longer feel the need to purchase birthday or congratulations cards along with my sauvignon blanc to make the clerks think I was buying wine for someone else. Or make sure I went to a different clerk each time. The coup de grace was telling the clerk all about the night's social event I had planned when it was really only a party for one. A friend in recovery called this behavior the "liquor store juggle."

***

I don't have to call the people I was with the night before and "fish" around for details on my behavior to fill in the gaps I couldn't remember.

***

I can skip walking the hallways of hotels in which I'm staying, searching for a trash bin where I can throw away my night-before-bottle-of-wine, so the staff won't know I drank it all by myself. Why did that even matter? Crazy making.

***

I no longer drink a half bottle of wine followed by chewing an entire package of gum before I go to a social event. Not sure when this ritual of pre-drinking began, but I'm sure people were on to me (as my daughter certainly was).

***

I am sitting here in the lobby sipping on a Clausthaler AF beer at the Hilton Garden in Fort Worth after the Sober Sis Retreat Dinner at Brewed Restaurant, where we had a mocktail tasting, a great meal, and an Enneagram presentation. Such strange feelings being at a social event and not drinking alcohol. I wonder what the hotel staff think about a group of teetotaling women. I'm not sure how I feel about it. One minute I am caught up in the excitement of Sober Sis, the possibilities, and all the amazing women here. The next minute I'm grieving my old best friend, sauvignon blanc. I don't know how to BE in this sober world. It feels awkward and strange. I wonder what my new path will look like.

***

It never gets old waking up clearheaded, hangover free, no regrets, no shame, and ready to start my day.

"No one ever wakes up in the morning wishing that they drank the night before." [6] —Jenn Kautsch/SoberSis

***

Sobriety has not helped me to be physically braver. I still have a complete fear of heights. Therefore, I have no desire to jump out of airplanes, bungee jump, or walk out on that clear plexiglass horseshoe thingy that hangs out over the Grand Canyon. Sobriety has changed none of that.

***

I find myself wanting to talk all the time about my sobriety. When I start to talk to Paul about it, his eyes glaze over. It's only been a little over a hundred days and talking about it makes him super uncomfortable. If I mention I miss having a glass of wine or a cocktail, I read total panic on his face. His financial analyst mind thinks I should just be done with it and put all things alcohol out of my mind, never to think about it again.

I put Paul through so much. And I cannot expect a normal drinker to possibly know what it's like to be me or how important it is to keep talking about it.

***

For the first time in many years, I could look my new doctor in the eye and tell her the truth about how much I drink. Absolutely nothing! I don't drink! Yay! It feels so liberating. Made my day …

***

I am 15 pounds lighter because I'm discovering there is an entire world beyond coming home from work and opening that bottle.

***

I no longer get irritated at the checker at Target, who asks this 68-year-old for her ID to purchase wine. And my world has opened up now that I have the choice to go through self-checkout.

***

I have been taking fancy Epsom salt baths with eucalyptus, rosemary, lavender, and peppermint (my absolute favorite), followed by my Insight Timer meditation app. I still miss my wine, but the cravings are less intense and they don't last as long.

***

I don't have to take a trip to the ATM to make sure I have cash hidden away in my wallet for impromptu wine purchases, or to separately pay for wine so that it doesn't show up on my grocery receipts.

***

Part of my job is to teach and coach social workers how to work with families who struggle with addiction. Isn't it crazy that so many of us in the recovery community are connected to teaching, coaching, nursing, wellness, and other related helping professions? I now stand in front of the class (as I will this morning) completely present and proud, without the cognitive dissonance of the past.

***

Gone is the shame of coming across empty wine bottles I forgot I hid in suitcases, or in boxes of holiday decorations, because I didn't want my husband to know. OMG, who was this person?

***

At three and a half months sober, I finally got up the nerve to tell my friend Susan I stopped drinking, and why. She sent me this text: "I am so honored that you shared this with me. I definitely have experienced a difference with you. I applaud your courage and strength. The most beautiful element of this equation is not only how your life will be enriched, but also the impact you will have on others. I LOVE IT! I love you and am very proud of you!"

***

"Drunk orders" from Amazon have ceased. And Lindsay now has a harder time sneaking stuff into my cart, thinking I won't notice when I push the order button. Another reason my financial analyst husband is happy with my new alcohol-free lifestyle. Unfortunately, now when a package arrives these days and I can't remember what I ordered, it's a little disconcerting to know that I no longer have the alcohol to blame!

***

I have become very aware of the vast difference in interpretations between: "Geez, you were pretty hilarious last night". Really? Was I? Because I don't even remember a thing about last night, versus: "I haven't had that much fun in ages! Loved being with you. I laughed so hard my stomach hurt. You were hilarious last night!" I was totally present and remembered it all.

***

I can put my eyeliner on straight. Well, straighter.

***

My restaurant checks have been cut in half, and in most cases, more than that. In almost any restaurant, my sauvignon blanc cost an average of $16 per glass. And of course, I can't recall a time I had just one glass. Interesting that wait staff never come back and ask you if you'd like another appetizer or main course, but: "Another glass of wine?" Fill-er up.

***

I have stopped "pairing" sauvignon blanc with decorating for the holidays. This Halloween was my first sober decorating activity since my last day one. This wine pairing has actually been one of my happy drinking memories, and—I'm not going to lie—this will be one tradition that I'll miss.

***

I really have so much more time in a day now that I'm not wasting time thinking about buying wine, drinking it, and the not-wanting-to-do-anything that follows, including the post-drinking cover-up. This is what freedom feels like.

***

Today marks four months for me. There are just no words to explain how much my Sober Sis Marco group means to me. (Giant tears running down my face.) Jenn, Ashley, Audrey, Beka, Cindy, Colleen, Ellen, Jan, Jane, Janet, Joy, Julann, Karen, Kelly, Laura, Dolores, Lindsay, and Robin. I would not be where I am today without you. And a heart-felt thanks to all the new friends I made at the Sober Sis retreat in Fort Worth.

***

I was cleaning and organizing my closet today and found my driver's license I lost last year. I can't tell you how many times I lost my license or credit card and had to order new ones because I had no idea where I put them. I can tell you what a stress reducer it is to know that they will be in the same place when I need them now.

***

I can write a check, send a card, make a list, journal, or write on chart paper in my classes and my handwriting is back to its pre-drinking, kindergarten teacher-like penmanship. Not one little shaky word, punctuation, or number.

***

My little brother (well, little to me—he is 57) told me last week that he looks forward to our conversations now because I have stopped repeating stuff over and over. And I thought I was just being such a brilliant, clever, and hilarious big sister.

***

I no longer have to say "I bruise easily" after waking up with unexplained cuts and bruises. Looking back, shouldn't that have been incentive enough to question my relationship with wine?

"The bottom is just the point where you begin to tell the truth." [7] —Tabitha Vidaurri

***

Lots of my sober friends have downloaded drinking apps to track their AF days and the money they have saved. I can't bring myself to do that because I don't want anyone to know how much I was drinking. And I really haven't saved much money because my new healthy addiction is fancy sparkling water and zero-proof spirits which cost nearly as much as my wine.

***

I have journaled every single day since my decision to stop the insanity. I started journaling many times in the past, but never stuck with it. I cannot tell you how putting my daily thoughts down on paper has become such an integral piece of my sober journey.

"Journaling is like whispering to oneself and listening at the same time." [8] —Mina Murray

***

I was never pulled over for driving under the influence. I certainly could have been. So many times. My drinking didn't jeopardize my career. I didn't lose any friendships because of my drinking; in fact, they always seemed to make excuses for me. When I came dangerously close to losing my marriage, my relationship with my daughter, and ultimately my grandchildren, that was all the incentive I needed. That was my tipping point. The cost of drinking had become too high a price to pay.

***

I am ridiculously passionate about teaching, and my evaluations reflect that. However, being AF allows me to be even more present. Last Friday, one of my students wrote: "I always love having you as an instructor, but today I really wanted to thank you for quieting down that noisy table. I could actually learn for the first time in six months of training." I wasn't always so in tune to my classroom when I came to teach hungover and sleep deprived. I'm so grateful I had this opportunity.

***

Today I tossed, canceled, or deleted all things vino: wine clubs, corks, charms, hats, T-shirts, Christmas ornaments (I was so proud of those sauvignon blanc and cabernet bottles inside blown glass), apps, books, cards, magnets, Pinterest pages, coolers, plaques. I am hanging on to the wine racks (they make exceptional towel holders) and the glasses (for guests and my new AF drinks).

***

I looked at myself in the mirror this morning and I really noticed how clear my skin looks, how bright my eyes are, how the bags under my eyes have practically vanished, and how my hair looks thicker and shinier. I literally said out loud: "Wow! I LOVE THIS WOMAN!" The final score? Love 1. Guilt & Shame 0. I finally passed the mirror test.

***

I find myself no longer trying to be everything to everyone. I heard someone say in a meeting that their original drug of choice was acceptance. That was me. I didn't know where someone else ended and I began. Boundaries were often nonexistent. I'm learning to lean out purposefully by walking away from things not meant for me.

I'm about two thirds of the way through Annie Grace's 100 Day Challenge. I am discovering that so much of my drinking resulted from surrendering or giving in to what other people want me to be or do, at the price of my own core values. I am not so naive as to think I only need to do things that make me happy, but so many times I "went along" just to keep the peace which left me RAW (resentful, angry, and wanting wine). I am CHOOSING to stay home for Thanksgiving.

Being AF has allowed me to speak up for myself and only do the things that support my sobriety. Haha. I'm quite sure Paul wonders who he is married to right now.

37

***

WARNING: Being alcohol free may significantly lower anxiety in your partner and, as a result, you may receive compliments and words of support. Paul just said, "You are my morning Peggi all the time now. What joy that is to me." I'm not exactly sure what that means, but I'll take it.

This side effect may feel strange and completely foreign at first. Should this behavior last for over four hours, don't consult with your physician. Count your blessings.

***

This will be my first alcohol-free Thanksgiving in years. My adult kids and grandkids will be at their dad's. Paul is going solo to his sister's house with my blessing. I have plans to go up to our cabin in the mountains for self-reflection and self-care. I am giving myself permission to be selfish about my sobriety. Snow is forecast. My dreaded moose furniture will keep me company.

***

We often see posts on public Facebook pages portraying "perfect lives," and it can sometimes make us feel we fall short, but this isn't the case on the Sober Sis and "We Are the Luckiest" Facebook pages. Members celebrate every sober success, big and small. And there is so much support when people struggle. There is such an overwhelming comfort in the ability to be raw and honest in this truly judgment-free zone. Nothing can replace the intimacy, the transparency, and the LOVE in these sobriety communities.

***

Recently, my university director asked me to take on a curriculum development project which is (as she knew) totally out of my comfort zone. Pre-AF, I would have likely been hungover, but not now. I could clearly envision how the work could be accomplished. Yesterday, I sat down and nearly completed the entire revision. This was big for me! I enjoyed the challenge, instead of fearing it.

***

For the first time in many years, I woke up this Thanksgiving morning with a smile on my face … no dread of what the day had in store, the glasses of wine I would drink at my sister-in-law's house just so I wouldn't feel lonely and think about how much I missed my own family. I can just envision how I'm going to feel tomorrow morning when I wake up without a hangover, remembering the entire day. And I won't be jeopardizing my life or others' driving home when I have no business getting behind the wheel.

***

I don't think I have had a hangover-free day-after-Thanksgiving morning in years. I'm sitting here, coffee in hand, reflecting that alcohol had been a part of Thanksgiving dating back to my childhood. There were huge family gatherings. I never liked them much. I'm sure that was because the evenings would end up with my parents fighting on the way or when we got home.

I also thought of the PTSD my cousins and I developed because of the mountains of dishes, pots, and pans we had to wash after dinner. It's a wonder we didn't become juvenile drinkers. What a nightmare. There were no non-stick pans, dishwashers, or disposals, and it literally took hours to do the clean-up. It wrinkled our fingers for days. In hindsight, a call to CPS [Child Protective Services] was probably warranted.

***

I still rejoice that I woke up yesterday without a hangover. Even my husband, who has no issues with alcohol, avoided his annual post-Thanksgiving hangover by choosing to skip the traditional overindulgence in Irish whiskey with his sisters. It's like we were both gifted with an extra day this year.

***

Two words: Topo Chico. Three words: Topo Chico-Lime.

***

I no longer have "drinking on the brain." I didn't realize just how much time was stolen from my life as I was thinking and bargaining with myself about drinking—when to drink, how much to drink, promising not to drink, where to stop and shop to drink, who I can drink with (oh, wait … that was mostly just me, because toward the end, I tried to hide my problem by drinking alone), promising to only drink on/at certain days/times/events, feeling the deep shame about my drinking … ugh … it was all so painful and exhausting. My personal Groundhog Day.

***

It's becoming more and more common now for me to break out in smiles FANAR (for absolutely no apparent reason). I kind of like it. Of course, people stay away from me when I do that, and that's just fine.

***

I have my sewing/quilting mojo back. I finished a quilt I had been working on for two years for my son Brett and made six Christmas stockings for my daughter's family. I hated the quilt I made for Brett—there were so many mistakes in it because I sewed half of it buzzed on wine. As a part of my healing, I knew I needed to finish the damn thing. I used to sew all the time before my love/hate affair with sauvignon blanc. What passion will you re-ignite with your alcohol-free life?

***

The words my daughter spoke gave me the excuse I needed to quit drinking. She stopped me from completely turning into my mother. I hope my new life will prevent Matt, Lindsay, and Brett from carrying my issues into their adulthood, keeping them out of recovery rooms and blaming their mother for their own issues with alcohol. I want them to be proud of how I overcame the one thing that was keeping me from being the mother and grandmother they deserve.

***

I wrote out my Christmas cards yesterday, and it reminded me of how many times over the past few years that my hands would shake when I was writing. Uncomfortably so. I used to make the excuse that I had too much caffeine. (I only drank one cup a day; on rare occasions, maybe two.) There would be times when I would have to hold one hand down with the other just to write a sentence. No rock bottoms here.

40

THIS SIDE OF ALCOHOL

***

Should I be worried that when a sister (what we fellow Sober Sis members call each other) posts a Marco video, I find myself talking to her out loud? Blowing kisses, reaching out and touching the screen with my hand? Answering, commenting, even though she can't hear or see me? Asking for a friend. There must be a diagnosis for that. Seriously, I thought these connections would be supportive, but they are so much more than that. It's impossible to put into words how deep these friendships go and how they reach so far beyond alcohol. I love that alcohol isn't the only thing we talk about anymore.

***

Lindsay called last night, and I noticed how much easier and lighter our conversation has become. She calls more often; she shares more of what's going on with her; she asks more questions and seems genuinely interested in what's happening in my life AND she doesn't get irritated because I now actually remember most conversations we've already had.

***

I never thought in a million years that I would ever be into meditation. I took a Personal Psychology class many, many years ago in college. The professor put a mantra on the chalkboard. (Yes; I am THAT old.) I had absolutely no idea what a mantra was. I thought it was a word scramble and tried to "solve the puzzle." He said that was the first time in thirty years of teaching that anyone tried to do that. Thank you, thank you. Anyway, meditation is now part of my daily routine. It allows me to have a space between my thoughts and my actions, allowing me to be more present.

***

Yesterday, my friend Janet and I were talking about how being AF for the holidays has been so calming—everything is simpler, slowed down, and less anxiety-provoking. This year, I'm mindfully choosing traditions to keep and some to lose that no longer serve me or my family or take away from the season's true meaning. This year, I gave myself permission to not spend days baking and frosting cookies, something I HAD to do in the past.

***

Last night, I had a wonderful evening with my 32-year-old colleague Liz, going to Thai and watching Frozen II. (BTW, so good, and we were the only two people in the theater.) Grand company, great conversation. I love that a young person wanted to hang out with this senior. If I was still drinking, I would have made excuses not to go so that I could go back to the hotel room and have my bottle of wine. I would have missed the opportunity to make a new friend. How many opportunities have I missed in the past?

***

My job as a trainer/coach for a local university requires a ton of traveling. Before becoming AF, I left so many things in my hotel rooms due to post-wine-morning brain fog. Pillows, clothes, Invisaligns, jewelry, contacts, and a record number of phone chargers, more than I could count. I can't even think about how much money I wasted, or how challenging it was to teach with a low-grade hangover the next day. Now I enjoy a spa, movie, Chinese food (my husband isn't a fan), take a walk and explore the area, connect with friends, or just be. And I don't leave shit behind.

***

We had the two sets of twin grandkids over for the weekend. I noticed how much more relaxed my husband was around them now that I'm not drinking. He pitched in more to help, and we both had a ton of extra patience. The kids were so affectionate (but seriously loud with their high-pitched voices) and there was no tension in the room caused by arguments we got into the night before because of my drinking. I wasn't full of shame and guilt. I kind of like this sobriety thing.

***

I had dinner last night with one of my best friends at a favorite Asian bistro. We had so much fun and laughed so hard our stomachs ached. I never imagined it was possible to have this much fun sans alcohol. And I cannot believe how the food tasted; it's like I'm growing new tastebuds. We then drove around the "Fabulous 40s,"

42

an area in Sacramento famous for their Christmas decorations, each massive street having their own holiday theme. One street was lined with luminaries for blocks. It was stunning. Being sober is like being reborn and looking at everything for the first time.

***

I no longer invite people over after having too much to drink, forget I did, and then get a phone call, asking what time they should come over and what should they bring. Sometimes a friend would ask me if I remembered inviting her. (Wow, that last part was hard to write–shame leaking everywhere.) The look on my face would reveal the answer.

***

My work has the most annoying, complicated system for travel reimbursement. Pre-sobriety, I would drink wine to reward myself for the torture it was to enter my expenses. As you might guess, entering information into a complex program while drinking wine is not a recipe for accuracy. Dare I say it's completely inversely related. Who knew?

***

Although it has been amazing to be sober for over five months with my children counted among my biggest supporters, the holidays have me reflecting on all the havoc and hurt my drinking caused them over the last ten years. There is still so, so much to repair. I pray that God gives me the time in which to do it.

***

Who would have ever thought that on July 12, 2019, I would introduce myself to 26 strangers in my Sober Sis Marco group, women from all over the country, from all backgrounds, who wanted to change their relationship with alcohol? Scared out of my mind, I was feeling so completely sad, full of shame, guilt, remorse, self-hatred, and defeat, and was experiencing incredible emotional pain. I was physically sick. I felt broken. I took a screenshot of myself that day and it's still so hard to look at it. It is, however, a reminder that I am no longer her.

Community is the backbone of recovery. We may initiate recovery in treatment, but lasting recovery only happens in community.

***

Now, on December 23, I am waking up in a house in Vero Beach, Florida, that belongs to one of my sober sisters. I'm celebrating my first alcohol-free Christmas holiday in years. I'm so grateful we can get away and do something completely different from our normal routine. I have been able to walk on the beach every day. Paul has been cycling up and down the A1. We have gone on many road trips exploring this beautiful Atlantic coastline. Life is good.

***

Tomorrow will be my first alcohol-free Christmas in years. I'll wake up tomorrow morning remembering everything about this Christmas Eve. We took a walk this evening where palm trees are wrapped in tiny white twinkling lights. I am honoring my family, my friends, my sober community, myself, and most of all, I am honoring Christ and the true meaning of Christmas. (Wow. I'm pretty choked up with emotion right now.) Sobriety is the gift that keeps on giving.

***

It's Christmas morning. I am totally present, hangover free, loving life in Vero Beach with Paul and my cup of Kona coffee. I highly recommend changing it up for the holidays in year one of sobriety. We have never gone away for the Christmas and New Year's (except for that one magical time that Paul was working in Aruba). Walking on the beach in the middle of winter is invigorating. Doing it sober is extraordinary.

***

In the first four decades of my life, drinking alcohol just wasn't anything I wanted to do on a regular basis. I was more interested in collecting beautiful liquor bottles to display on my new buffet. Then my fifties hit, and the switch flipped. Wine became my go to during the end of my career as a county social worker in child welfare, where I experienced secondary trauma, an extremely toxic work environment, and an unfortunate situation where I ended up as a whistleblower. My stomach hurt every time I walked into the office, eight hours a day, for two whole years. Wine seemed to be the antidote, making it all go away for a few hours each night. I use those experiences in my current position, passionately teaching new social workers to make sure they take the time out for self-care while working in a rewarding, but much under-appreciated and trauma-producing profession.

***

I am acutely aware of how isolated I had become because of my drinking. My world had become so small. I am just reconnecting with a few friends, trusting some of them enough to share what I'm going through. Most are genuinely happy for me. Some, I'm sure, think it's just another phase … They have seen me "take breaks" from alcohol before. The majority are seriously surprised alcohol was a serious problem for me, reminding me of the energy it sucked from me to hide it. For some others, there is nothing we have in common anymore. And that's okay.

***

Yesterday, I was feeling melancholy about my sober journey. I was full of a sadness I couldn't name. In being fully present, I'm looking more into my family of origin for answers. I thought about my mother, who was so creative and talented, who, at one time, decorated windows for Christmas in a downtown department store. Yet my brothers and I never knew what mom we were going to get when we walked in the door—our happy mom or the withdrawn, not-so-nice one. I didn't know until early adulthood that my mother's behavior was largely because of drinking. It was all so confusing. Dying at 51, she never had the chance to take control and heal. I am so grateful that I do.

***

The Advil people must not be fans of the sober-minded movement. My Advil intake has practically dropped to zero since I quit drinking.

***

When I drank wine, I had a habit of not eating or eating very little … a dead giveaway to my family that I HBD (Had been drinking).

***

As the New Year approaches, I'm coming to terms with the fact that I can't take back the pain I caused others because of my drinking. I know I have become a better person and that feels good, so authentic. I also realize that I have no control over when, if, or how people will choose to forgive me.

45

***

As I move closer to 2020 [Ed. note: Little did I know what a shit show that was going to be!], I am committed and excited to be on track to be alcohol free for the entire year. I'll do everything it takes to make that happen.

***

2019 was the year I stopped making and breaking resolutions. I have been alcohol free for almost six months. For those of you who are new in your sober journey, always remember that alcohol will never change. It will always be a wolf in sheep's clothing. There will always be new marketing ploys that will try to pull you back in, to make you think that New Year's without a champagne toast is criminal. Happy New Year! May you have 2020 vision (haha) all year long.

***

Today I got to meet and spend time with my new sober friends Jan and her husband, George, whose home we were staying in for the holidays. Jan summed up our almost six months of sobriety in the way only she could: "We were intelligent women who just happen to be walking down the alcohol path together ... it's a good thing we are so fucking smart! We recognized it before it became an unmanageable maze." LOVE THIS WOMAN!

***

My first sober vacay ended with a day of extreme challenges. I left my wallet at Jan's, my luggage fell out of our SUV on the side of I-95 (don't ask), I cracked the glass on my iPhone by sitting on it while at the rest stop, and, when we arrived at the airport, I realized I'd booked two different second leg flights for Paul and me. Pre-sobriety, I would have lost it completely and had copious amounts of wine in the airport bar. Nope. After getting really pissed off at each other, fixing the flights, we got over it and talked about how amazing our trip was.

***

I believed that drinking wine made me more fun, more joyful, more introspective. While under the influence, I was sure I could solve every world problem that existed (not that I could remember the next day any of the solutions I came up with). I certainly wasn't fun, joyful, or introspective. I was merely taking a holiday from mindfulness.

***

Having been cursed with extremely poor vision, I can now report that I don't have trouble putting in my contacts in the morning anymore! This is so big for me! My eyes used to get really, really dry after a night of sauvignon blanc. Most of the time, my hands would also shake, making contact insertion challenging. The panic attacks I would have if I couldn't get them in were only matched by the panic attacks I would have because I couldn't get them out, after drinking and falling asleep with them in.

Chapter Five

I'm getting there
(Six to 12 months)

"Some people can hold their breath underwater
for over three minutes.
Some people can go out for one drink and be satisfied.
I can do neither."
—Alicia Gilbert

My heart is so happy to write that, today, I have been alcohol free for 180 days! To me, 180 implies that I have done an about-face, completely turning my life around, facing in the opposite direction from where I used to be.

***

I just spent six days at the cabin on a purposeful, intentional self-retreat. I appreciate Paul's understanding of how much I needed this. I loved the company and the conversations.

Reflection Day 1
Something noticeably gone from my alcohol-free life—I was taking a hot shower this morning, thinking back to all those times I showered with my head leaning against the tiled wall because I was so hungover it felt like my hair hurt.

Reflection Day 2

My oldest son, Matt, turns 40 today. How is that even possible? What better way to honor him (and Lindsay and Brett) than to be simultaneously celebrating my six-month soberversary with him? On to the next milestone, July 12, when it will be one year.

Reflection Day 3

I listen to music each morning now without that disgusting gag-while-I-brush-my-teeth thingy I constantly experienced after a night of drinking wine. I sometimes even dance like no one's watching. They say that's what I'm supposed to do, right?

Reflection Day 4:

I am sitting in bed, under my weighted blanket (my favorite Christmas present), hands (not shaking) wrapped around a steaming cup of Kona Sunrise coffee, watching the sun rise over a blanket of undisturbed snow. It's so quiet. I thank God I am seeing, feeling, and tasting all of this through my new lens of sobriety.

Reflection Day 5

Regardless of what you may have heard, there is no deadline to take down the Christmas tree. We were away for two weeks, and I haven't had enough time to enjoy my decorated-while-sober tree. My tree, my rules. So, talk away, neighbors, about that crazy lady who still has her tree up. They just don't know that every ornament, every tiny light, reflects how far I have come this year.

Reflection Day 6:

Besides Advil, there are more companies who may not be celebrating my sober lifestyle: Pepto-Bismol, Tums, Rolaids, Alka-Seltzer, Zantac, Pepcid AC. I'm sure there are others. All that time, I blamed my abdominal issues on stress and food "not agreeing with me"—when, in reality, it was my body begging me to stop drinking wine.

***

I now actually DO the items on my "to do" list (which used to make me feel overwhelmed and want to drink). I feel good at the end of the day, knowing I have accomplished or made progress on most listed tasks. I sleep better. I'm less stressed. Add these to my "so many benefits of leading a sober life."

***

One of our sober sisters posted about "Be the Sugar" at her school—i.e., when you practice kindness, you start seeing it everywhere. Well, I had it slightly wrong this past week and was practicing "Eat the Sugar." Geez, this is a switch because in the past I used to always opt to "Drink the Wine."

I had never really been into sweet things before. Turns out I'm not the only one. It's a well-reported phenomenon that some people who quit the booze find themselves reaching for the sweet stuff. Both alcohol and sugar boost our dopamine levels. Dopamine is the "reward" chemical in the brain. So, this week, I am committing to be, not eat, the sugar.

***

I was 30,000 feet in the air last night, sitting in a completely full Southwest plane, tired from work and traveling, and this random thought came across my mind and made me smile: I no longer must worry that while I'm gone, my husband might run across wine bottles I had no memory of hiding around the house.

***

I can feel how relaxed by husband and my adult children are around me now. This is so big because no one ever knew what was going to happen when I started drinking, especially me. I was so completely unpredictable. I could be absolutely fine, or I wasn't. I was oblivious to the hurt and pain I was causing.

***

While I was in San Diego for a training, I went to dinner with my co-workers and my cousin, Russ, to a beautiful restaurant in Balboa Park, The Prado. They had two glasses of wine. I had two glasses of club soda with pomegranate puree with a squeeze of lime. Their checks were $72 each, mine was $40. Boom.

***

My sister-in-law invited us to watch the Super Bowl. (The members of my husband's family are huge 49er fans.) I gave myself permission NOT to go. Laura McKowen writes about being able to turn down activities that might contribute to relapse:

> "...needing safety, space and the 'simplicity' of just being without having to fight against the tide ... giving myself a chance." [9]

The hubs isn't thrilled with my choice, but he is respecting it.

***

I owe so much of my continued sobriety to my Sober Sis and We Are the Luckiest communities. Hearing of other people's successes and of how their lives have improved keeps me inspired to continue on my own sober path. It also gives me opportunities to support others who are struggling. These support groups have given me and others the courage to be open and honest, which is an essential component of healing from addiction.

***

A very simple "Aha!" moment for me: I started drinking several years ago to not feel pain and now I realize that, all along, alcohol was the pain. Deep thought, but true.

***

Today, I am reflecting on how the support of the recovery community is critical to maintaining my sobriety. My husband says he is very proud of me, but he isn't really that interested in talking about it. I published an article about *Rethinking Drinking* in an East Coast women's magazine over a month ago, and he has never asked to read it. Sometimes I feel like my own island—not sad, really, maybe disconnected? People who have never had issues with alcohol cannot understand.

***

Last night was BIG. My friend Linda W and I had dinner at the Echo & Rig, Butcher, Steakhouse in Downtown Sacramento. We ran into some old friends who told me I looked great. I felt great. After dinner, Linda and I attended the Cirque du Soleil performance of Amaluna. We splurged by buying VIP tickets and had access to the Hennessy Brandy sponsored VIP tent where food and spirits were abundant and free. This was my first social outing since I have become AF. I witnessed many people get loud and obnoxious (so many of them with their kids in tow). Loved the food, passed on the booze. It was a lot easier than I thought.

***

Hitting the double century, marking 200 days of sobriety, is reason to be happy; but truth be told, I still feel the loss and I gotta be REAL. I still miss drinking sometimes. I still have why-can't-I-drink-like-a-normal-person? thoughts. Long streaks of sobriety aren't a ticket to freedom. Big milestones can be both a reason to celebrate and a bit of a trigger. So, today, I am mindfully renewing my commitment to continue my alcohol-free journey.

***

There is still so much to heal between my husband and me, but there is a huge sense of peace and trust that hasn't been in our marriage, our home, for several years.

> "Being in a relationship with someone who drinks too much is a lot like living with infidelity. It's no different from your partner having a lover, except the lover isn't another person but a thing." [10] —Laura McKowen

I have met and talked with several women who have told me that their partners thought they were having an affair when, all along, it was alcohol.

***

I have a couple family members who cannot believe I became sober by enrolling in "some online program she found on Facebook that only cost a little less than a hundred dollars." One of them told my husband she researched Sober Sis and found it to be lacking. These two have expressed their collective opinion (not to me, of course), that my sobriety cannot last without a "more serious and intensive intervention." Fortunately, I know better, have trust in myself, and continue to surround myself with friends and family who choose to be on Team Peggi.

✲✲✲

Ugh, I replaced my bed mattress pad yesterday morning and came face to face with a GIANT red wine stain that I totally forgot about. For a minute, it brought back a not-so-great memory of falling asleep with a wine glass in my hand, waking up to ruined sheets and a carpet stain I blamed on my grandkid's prune juice. I rarely drank red wine because I didn't like it. I only drank red wine when there was nothing else. Shame crept in. (Ugh, shame is such a continuing theme running through my story.) So, I flipped the damn mattress over and smiled.

✲✲✲

Like so many of you, I blamed myself daily, sometimes hourly (so did my family), for not being able to control my drinking. Not. Any. More. Holly Whitaker writes in her book *Quit Like A Woman*:

> "It's the same as saying it's not the alcohol's fault, it's YOURS you can't do it right. [This] is the same as blaming the homeless man for his lack of home, the single mom on welfare for her lack of ambition, the battered wife for staying." [11]

Thank God for writers like Holly who help us, and those who judge us, to reframe our lenses. Powerful words.

✲✲✲

My "appearances" on Marco Polo have made me much more self-confident and a better public speaker. If I can "show up" with no makeup, my coke-bottle glasses and complete bed head, and not be self-conscious, I can do ANYTHING. How much more real can I get?

***

It never gets old that I now have five to six more hours in the day when I can be productive—walking sewing, reading, studying, watching a complete TV episode and being able to remember it! I have time for meditating, taking a bath, or just having a conversation with a friend. After drinking that first and second and third—okay, sometimes fourth—glass of wine at five o'clock, I stopped living my life until the next day when it started all over again.

***

Yesterday, I stopped at a gas station near my home and when I pulled up to the pump, I experienced a flash-of-shame attack. My mind went to a memory of how many times I tossed empty wine bottles in the trash there so no one would find them in the bin at home. I often wondered if I was on video camera doing that. Just as quickly, I forgave myself because I am not that person anymore.

***

I'm choosing not to have anyone in my life right now who isn't fully supportive of the person I am becoming. To be fair, I'm still very selective about who I choose to share my journey with. Not everyone deserves to be in my life right now. I call it "regulating the space around my heart."

***

I am learning to appreciate the difference between isolation and solitude. Isolation, aka loneliness, happens when we negatively react to our environment and surroundings. I know that I can be in a room full of people and feel completely alone. I used drinking to combat that lonely, "not fitting in" feeling. Solitude is taking time out to recharge my batteries so that I can be my "best self" when I head back out into this crazy world.

***

Hangover-free mornings give me the opportunity to pay it forward by writing encouraging words or by cheering on people in the recovery community. I also LOVE to send hand-written cards for birthdays and for "just because." TJ Max and Home Goods have great cards that don't cost as much as a bottle of wine! I stock up regularly.

***

Yesterday, I spent the day with several Sober Sis women. We had lunch at an amazing restaurant, August 1 Five (great food and mocktail menu, by the way), in downtown San Francisco, followed by a walk across the street to Books Inc. where we sat and listened to Laura McKowen read my favorite excerpt from her recently released book *We Are the Luckiest*:

> "As I sat there crying, I remembered something from years ago, before Alma, before any of this. It was the end of a long day of my first yoga teacher training, and we were all gathered in a circle, asking questions, discussing the day. One of the students raised his hand and said, matter-of-factly, 'I'm afraid I can't stop drinking.'
>
> The room went silent. All of our eyes went to our teacher, David.
>
> Without missing a beat, he smiled, looked at him, and said, 'Of course you can. Are you drinking right now?'
>
> 'No.'
>
> 'And now?'
>
> He smiled and said softly, 'No.'
>
> '... and how about right now?'
>
> We all smiled this time.
>
> 'No.'" [12]

This passage had a profound impact on my sobriety. A lightbulb went on. I didn't have to think in terms of forever. Whenever I think I just can't do this, that I can't possibly be AF for the rest of my life, I read this passage. I am not drinking now.

***

During my drinking days, I was always afraid of saying things to people I didn't mean. Now I'm even more afraid I might say things

55

I do mean. I'm trying to rein in some of those truth bombs that seem to fly out my mouth.

***

I MAY have had a conversation last week with some ladies about drinking a bottle of wine and then replacing it with water and food coloring so my husband wouldn't know I drank the whole damn bottle. Geez, drinking and covering it up became close to a full-time job, so all-consuming and exhausting. I am now using my evil for good.

***

Today, I'm celebrating the number 7. Why do I find this number so fascinating? Well, there are 7 days of the week, 7 colors of the rainbow, 7 notes on the musical scale, 7 brides for 7 brothers (lame, I know), 007 (haha, love that one), and today marks 7 months that I have been alcohol free. It took a lot of hard work and tears, but I'm finding it to be easier every day.

***

I have a friend, Tami, spending the night with me at our cabin in Lake Almanor. Last night we had delicious salads, fancy sparkling water, a luxurious soak in the hot tub under a starry, starry, and more starry sky, followed by amazing conversation by the fire. I crawled into bed and slept so well. Sleep had been elusive when I was drinking. I woke up with a clear heart and mind. I remembered everything. Coffee this morning tasted like the most decadent dessert in a fancy restaurant. Glorious.

***

Driving myself to events, family gatherings (if I choose to attend), and leaving whenever I feel like it, has become one of my sober superpowers.

***

My son Brett called to talk about a job interview he was going to. He was really struggling between his appreciation of and loyalty to his current employer, and the opportunities he thought might be possible at the new company. I was fully present for him. One of my greatest joys of sobriety is the ability to totally "be there" for my kids (and myself).

***

I have given myself permission to say "no" next time I'm asked to be a designated driver. A couple days ago, I had the experience of going to dinner and watching a couple of sixty-somethings drink way too much. I then attempted and failed several times to convince them it was time to go home. In the car, I had to listen to them tell me over and over how much they loved me. (Geez, that used to be me.) It's time for me to choose my social outings more carefully. Another AFGO (According to Anne Lamott: Another Fucking Growth Opportunity).

***

I have so much more patience with the grandkids. We had four of them over this weekend. We did puzzles, art projects, walked, sledded, played games (they love "Headbands" and "Our Moments" conversation cards), took bubble baths, soaked in the hot tub, read books, and snuggled on the couch watching a movie by the fire. Faye asked, "Can I just live here?" (Haha, absolutely not.) My heart is full.

***

I really envy those who can moderate their drinking, but I know I'm not one of them. When I was drinking, I could never guarantee that "one or two drinks" would actually be "one or two drinks." In her blog, Katie Koschalk wrote:

> "I didn't want A drink, I wanted lots of drinks. [One drink] would be like having only one slice of pizza." [13]

We are all on different paths. As my friend Judy says, "My story isn't yours. Yours isn't mine. Ours aren't theirs."

***

More thoughts on why moderation isn't my path. I often used alcohol to deal with negative emotions, to numb myself, to not give a damn. I realize now that people who don't have issues with alcohol don't stay up at night wondering about whether they have a drinking problem or pondering if they should quit. They don't turn to alcohol when a relationship breaks up. Alcohol isn't part of their life enough to give it a thought. My friend Susan rarely, I mean rarely, has more than one or two drinks. That wasn't me. That was never me.

***

Hmmm, today is National Margarita Day. For a mad minute, happy drinking memories popped into my head. But then I visualized the day my daughter looked at me with tears in her eyes telling me I needed to do something about my drinking. Those happy memories were exposed for what they really are—fiction.

***

Phew! We survived National Margarita Day. But now I feel inspired to find out who I might contact to establish/proclaim a "National Alcohol-is-no-longer-fucking-up-my-life Day." What do you think?

***

I find that one of my new sober superpowers is telling people about my choice to be alcohol free. It was hard at first. Brett told me I that I should tell people I trust. It took me almost four months to tell my best friend. I do have varying degrees of telling, from I-did-a-reset-and-I-felt-so-good-I-never-went-back, to sharing my bigger story. I'm still out in the world, teaching for a local university, but even with that, I hope that someday that won't even deter me. Many people are reluctant to tell others about their sober journey. I get that. For me, the telling makes it all that much more real and keeps the thoughts away that maybe I could ever go back to drinking.

***

The words we choose to describe people matter. I believe sincerely that labeling keeps us from seeing the person within. Rachel Hart talks about how labels reduce a complex, multifaceted person to a single behavior. If other people choose to call themselves "alcoholics" and they are comfortable with that, I have no issue. For me, personally, I would love to ditch that label entirely. I feel like it keeps me stuck in one chapter of a story, represents one small part of me, which no longer exists. My preferred labels, if I must have one, are "sober" (it took me time to feel comfortable with that one), "non-drinker," and "AF."

Oh, and because I choose not to drink the same substance that's used to fuel my car, I believe I can also label myself as "quite brilliant." Yes. That works.

***

Picture me, standing tall, feet apart, head up, chin up, hands on hips: "SOBRIETY DOES NOT DEFINE ME!" I am so much more than that. I am a mother, social worker, teacher, writer, wife, grandmother, friend, sister, auntie, cousin, daughter, quilter, mentor, coach, facilitator, justice fighter, and a lifelong learner. Now, sans alcohol, I just do these things so much better.

***

My daughter called yesterday and said: "Hey, Mom. I'm just calling you to tell you that there will be a lot of alcohol at Jason's birthday party so I thought you might feel more comfortable coming over on Sunday instead." Ugh. I felt like someone punched me in the heart. I know her call was coming from a good place with all good intentions, but how awful that I put her in a position where she felt she had to say that to me. Shame on (past) me.

***

One of my sober allies has become more aware of her friends' and family's drinking patterns and loves to "debrief" with me on her way home from events. Her observation this weekend was her friend's obsession with clean eating and exercise, who then proceeded to get blackout drunk both nights. She found it interesting that they consider this type of disparate behavior to be normal. Nothing to see here. Keep on walking.

***

Brett went on a date Wednesday night and I asked how it went:

> Brett: "It was okay, but she doesn't really drink, and she was buzzed after one."
> Me: "What if she didn't drink at all?"
> Brett: "That would be weird dating someone who doesn't drink." [Ed. note: Ouch.)
> Me: "Brett, you remember I stopped drinking, right?"
> Brett: "That's different."

The thing is, it was only last year when I thought the same way he did. I felt sorry for every person on the planet who didn't drink. I couldn't imagine living a life without alcohol in it. (I would miss out on so many things, like blackouts and hangovers.)

***

During my drinking days, if I saw that there was a "high wind warning" like last Friday (in California, it's synonymous with "super windy"—we are weather wimps), and admittedly, it was pretty nasty out there, I would easily convince myself that it was just too windy to walk and I would skip it. Now, I tell myself, "No problem, just think how many more calories you'll burn with the resistance."

***

I was walking in McKinley Park with Susan yesterday and she asked if I missed drinking. My mind flashed back to a time when Paul and I had good friends over for dinner. I got so drunk, I walked out into the garage, where the concrete floor seemed to rise up and smash me in the face before I passed out in a fetal position. "Not today," I answered.

***

Today, the memory of an old friend, Pops, crossed my mind. He was a former heroin user who had been sober for 30 years. I asked him what made him decide to stop using. He told me he had to steal every day to get the money to buy and use. Then he had to do it all over again the next day. He said using heroin became "just too damn much work" and so he got sober. I didn't steal to buy alcohol, but alcohol certainly stole from me. And it was a lot of work to keep up with the façade. Rest in peace, Pops.

***

I learned a new term this week, "emotional sobriety," which is being able to comfort oneself and cope with all the negative emotions that were ignored while drinking. Emotional sobriety requires the deeper work, the uncovering of all those underlying reasons we drink. Getting sober requires much more that stopping drinking. I liken it to the iceberg analogy. The part we see is our drinking behavior; what lies beneath the waterline are all the reasons we chose to poison our bodies with ethanol. So, along with the joyous, proud, and peaceful moments, I'm allowing myself to work through the feelings of fear, shame, isolation, pain, regret—all with the intention to create my best self.

***

After four challenging days of virtual teaching, followed by three days of babysitting the two sets of twin grandkids, an image of sitting down with a glorious cold glass of sauvignon blanc crossed my mind. Looking through my journal, I found this:

"The voice which tells you next time will be different should be avoided at all costs." [14]

Amen to that.

***

In the past, I justified my drinking by calling myself "high functioning." Functional drinkers make up about 20% of the US population. Many started problem drinking later in life like I did, work full time, and have stable relationships and high earnings. Well, nix the high earnings part—I am a social worker. By pure luck, I have never gotten a DUI. For at least the past five years, I convinced myself that I had control over my drinking. I successfully ignored, or made excuses for, the fights with my husband and the embarrassing incidents with my friends and family, until it was almost too late.

***

I woke up this morning thinking about the thousands of wine corks I used to collect in giant glass vases. (Come on, admit it: lots of you did, too.) Our neighbors did their whole bar backsplash with them. Early in our sobriety journey, my sober sis Kelly posted a video of ceremoniously dumping a giant glass jar of corks into the trash. All I know is that my trophy cork collection suffered when I switched to twist tops (when uncorking a bottle became, of course, much too time-consuming and inconvenient).

***

One of my sober sisters just returned from a week's vacay in Florida with lifelong friends. She was apprehensive about going because cocktails have been a central activity at their reunions.

When asked by one of her friends if she was ever going to drink again, Janet replied: "Why would I? Not drinking is my new superpower."

***

Just keeping it real today. It's interesting to me how reading other people's posts where they write about moderating, or attempting to moderate, keeps triggering something in me. There is no judgment. I am happy for them. My thoughts go to, "What's wrong with me that I can't do that?" Yet, intrinsically, I know that moderation isn't an option for me. That door has closed.

> "For me, it was all or nothing. I chose nothing, which in the end has turned out to be my all." [15] —Lucy Rocca

***

Thoughts on being eight months alcohol-free today. Any bad day sober has been better than my best day drinking. Not drinking feels like it's becoming my new normal. I'm grateful I have a job that enables me to have the resources to keep learning, digging deep, working hard to rewire my brain, setting goals, and actually meeting them. I continue to have my mind blown by the love and support of the Sober Sis and Luckiest Club communities.

***

Laura McKowen's words about COVID-19 are brilliant: "We are in a better place because we are sober. It may not feel like it, but listen, we can be present, clear, and we can make choices big and small that add value and not chaos.

Stress and fear happen when we feel a loss of control. It can feel disorienting and helpless. If you are putting in as much effort as you can to address COVID and are taking all the steps within your control to try to influence a positive outcome, you are doing as much as you can. Staying sober and present is within our control and keeps us available to help whenever and wherever we might be needed."

As I anticipate the cancellation of my classes, coaching, and my very first presentation at a national conference, I admit to feeling sorry for myself. I have a personality that thrives on being in the classroom with the students. Thank you, Laura, for reminding me that this is much bigger than me. Instead, I should ask: How can I help? What can I offer to support others in this tsunami of fear? Thank God I am sober and present to do just that.

***

I just want to throw this out there. I predict that one day "2020" will be synonymous with "mind-blowingly fucked up." Let's use it in a sentence: "Wow, that was really 2020, wasn't it?"

***

It doesn't matter if you are on Day 1, Day 21, Day 100, Day 365+. If you are doing things sober for the first time or the 1000th. If you drank yesterday or are a successful moderator. If you are 17 or 67. We all have something to teach each other. We all can lift each other up, not only during these crazy-ass times, but every day. People ahead of us in sobriety serve as mirrors of what we want to be.

***

Ah, I can't help but think that we humans are being tested with not only the pandemic, but now wildfires, floods, and politics. It has shaken our world. No longer can we assume and depend upon the comfort of safety, security, and unity. We can no longer take for granted the fact that schools and businesses will be open, that grocery store shelves will be stocked, that we can congregate in our houses of worship, that we can hug each other. With COVID, it has reduced us to our essential selves, and with that, what a gift it is to be alcohol free right now.

***

Now that I no longer get in a hot shower to lessen a hangover or lean my aching head on the shower wall while I'm shaking, gagging, and/or crying, taking a shower has become a favorite part of my morning. I love all the shower bombs out there; there are some for breathing, calming, sleeping, and headaches. I bought some loofa gloves (5 for 5 on Amazon) and I cannot tell you how alive my skin feels when I step out of that shower, ready to take on the new, albeit socially distanced, day.

63

***

During this incredibly unreal pandemic, I'm reminded of just how important it is to continue the work of emotional sobriety. From experience, it's easy to think I am "all better" and that I just might be able to drink like a normal person. I'm quite confident that that kind of thinking wouldn't end well for me. The pros of drinking are lies. I am recommitting to staying strong and stopping the energy-draining thought processes of how to keep this life-sucking substance in my life.

***

If COVID happened this time last year, I certainly wouldn't have been driving to Costco to pick up the suddenly elusive package of toilet paper. (I'm still clueless about what was behind that mass-hysteria reaction of hoarding TP for a pandemic that doesn't cause intestinal turbulence.) Nope, I would have been going to Costco to stock up on multiple bottles of my favorite sauvignon blanc, because wine would have trumped toilet paper, no matter what was going on in world events. The ride home would have comprised me drinking half a bottle and worrying about where I would hide the rest.

I also think I might have graduated to day drinking. It would have been a perfect time to check out.

> "The old me would have been giddy at the prospect of sheltering in place where I could drink myself into oblivion without any real-world obligations getting in the way." [16] —Alicia Gilbert/Soberish

What a frightening thought …

***

British journalist Johann Hari believes that humans become addicted to substances, not because of the pleasurable effects of the drugs, but because they feel disconnected from others. He believes that the opposite of addiction is connection. To be happy, humans need trust and emotional attachment. Hari's words resonated with me because I drank more when I felt disconnected from my husband and some of my family members. I felt even more disconnected when I found myself in the position of being a whistleblower at work and dealing with the bullying and ostracizing that followed. My husband, who has always worked in the private sector, criticized me for not standing up for myself, so I stopped talking to him about it. The amount of my drinking correlated with how disconnected I felt. I felt unworthy of connection. I was falling further and further into the abyss.

***

Yesterday someone said something that really stuck with me: "Drinking made things that were not okay, okay." It's worth repeating: "Drinking made things that were not okay, okay." This couldn't be any truer for me. When she said that, images immediately popped into my head: of driving after drinking, of telling my ex-director to "fuck off" at a restaurant (to this day, I cannot believe he forgave me), of hiding wine in my boots. Part of the work of sobriety is to unpack that shame we carry so that we can love ourselves again.

***

Finding the right people to tell is crucial to becoming and staying sober. Some people are uncomfortable talking about it. I found out right away that many people, including some of those closest to me, don't understand addiction. Why would they? Their lack of insight was sometimes painful. Yet I knew if I didn't tell people, I would leave that option open in my life where I could go back to thinking I could control my drinking. I cannot. You don't have to tell the world, but it's important to tell everything to at least one or two people, so that if you slip under the radar, they'll seek you out.

***

With the world so wonky right now, do any of you who are on a sober-minded path need a booster shot, an incentive, to stay the course? Go back and look at pictures of yourself pre and in early sobriety. For me, it was looking at my first video I posted in my Sober Sis Marco group, two days sober. It was so emotional—I saw a very sad, broken woman staring back at me. I was puffy, I had bags under my eyes, I looked like a deer in a headlight. I barely recognize her now. In the video, I said: "I think this Sober Sis thing is going to work." I was right.

***

One of the scariest, most anxiety-laden, and most shameful parts of drinking for me (so shameful, it has taken me over eight months to even talk about it) were the blackouts. You would think they might have made me seriously question my decision to continue putting poison in my body. But, no! Sarah Hepola's words hit home:

> "There is something fundamentally wrong with losing the narrative of your life." [17]

My blackouts hurt and embarrassed my family the most. I have all the risk factors for blackouts: a genetic predisposition for being able to hold my liquor, drinking quickly (especially when I started hiding my drinking), skipping meals, and being female. My friend Judy describes blackouts as "your personality totally extinguished for the night." Brilliant, as Judy often is. I'm proud to say I'm now a retired blackout artist.

***

For years, my husband made a habit of bringing me my Kona coffee in the morning, so on those days that he didn't, I knew I had royally screwed up the night before. (Black- or gray-outs would be the more honest descriptors.) My "hangxiety" would kick up into high gear. I would wait for him to say something, and if he didn't talk to me at all, I knew things were way worse than I thought. That morning coffee ritual has become the symbol of my sobriety. No more walks of shame to the coffeepot. Now the only reason he may not bring me coffee is that I have developed a habit of getting up early to write and journal, so I sometimes have to make my own coffee—a price I gladly and proudly pay. It's a reminder of the predictable life I have worked so hard to achieve.

***

I began this journey with a seemingly irreparable marriage. I put in many, many hours over the past nine months with the reset, online courses, Marcos, Zooms, "Lives," books, podcasts, blogs, meditation, mantras, journaling, a retreat, vision board, texts, therapy. I asked my husband, "Do you ever wonder who you are married to now?" He answered: "Not at all. You're the woman I fell in love with."

***

Upon hearing that our country is sheltering in place until April 30 (my daughter's 39th birthday) thanks to the pandemic, I'm feeling kind of heavy. (Thank God I didn't know the shelter in place would last far, far beyond April 30.) Weighted down. Paul went home for a couple days, so I'm alone in our cabin. I remembered the sign my friend Janet gave me for Christmas: "DANCE LIKE NO ONE IS WATCHING." There is such power in moving to the beat of music because it releases all those happy chemicals, particularly dopamine, oxytocin, serotonin, and endorphins. Dancing is one of the most effective tools for releasing negative emotions and replacing them with positive ones.

***

I am learning that sobriety, especially during these uncertain times of COVID, has given me the tools to get out of my head for a minute when things feel scary. I can breathe. I can look around. Where am I at this exact moment? Is what I am thinking the truth? Do I have everything I need? Are my children and my grandkids safe? Do I hear the birds singing? The ability to be present deflates the anxiety of future tripping.

***

Last year, I would have been center stage at all the COVID virtual happy hours that are now popping up everywhere. Any excuse to drink, right? Consider this: Majid Asgard, M.D., from Loyola University, writes:

> "Drinking can disrupt the body's ability to mount an adequate immune response to a stressful situation such as impeding a healthy response to the coronavirus … impairing signaling processes known as cytokine [which are] important fighters in the immune system's cellular arsenal." [18]

Knowing this is an incentive for me to stay sober because my age already puts me in the most vulnerable population for COVID.

***

For years, the alcohol industry has been bombarding all of our senses with information that romanticizes ethanol. You would expect nothing less during the pandemic. Meet the "Quarantini." With bars being closed across the country because of the coronavirus, the Quarantini was born from the idea that people need to create cocktails from whatever is in their liquor cabinet. There is no specific recipe. Perfect for consuming in isolation or via a virtual "happy hour" with similarly isolated friends. This cannot be a good sign ...

***

During this pandemic, my daughter somehow miraculously balances teaching 29 kindergarteners while juggling two sets of twins at home. How can a five-year-old learn anything in a virtual setting? I'm in awe of her.

I don't know how the social workers I teach can work to keep children safe when access to them is so limited. They are my heroes. How are social workers sleeping at night, while worrying about their caseloads and their own families, while also knowing full well that the school closures are contributing to more child abuse because the kids can't go to the one place, they feel safe—school.

COVID is scary, tragic, and devastating to so many, across all walks of life. Unlike so many others, I am fortunate that I'm still working and able to maintain my lifestyle. I know that the pandemic has been easier for me to handle because nothing in my life has been harder than getting sober. It has been the great preparer for any future challenge that will come my way.

***

I thought I had cleared out every alcohol-related item in my house, but as I was rearranging stuff in the kitchen yesterday, I came across a collection of wine stoppers. There, before me, were Mickey Mouse, beautiful blown glass, a silver Christmas deer head, and a hand-carved wooden heart, all from places we visited or that were received as gifts. Naturally, I don't think I ever used a single one of them, because whoever heard of having wine left in a bottle?

THIS SIDE OF ALCOHOL

✱✱✱

I can see where my drinking contributed to my "addiction" to chaos. Sadly, it became a way of life for me. Even though I had/have a very successful career and looked so together on the outside, I was a train wreck on the inside. Mark Griffiths, Ph.D., writes in his blog:

> "People are increasingly seduced into believing that intensity equals being alive. When that happens, the mind becomes wired for drama and the soul is starved of meaningful purpose." [19]

I could see this in the families and adults I worked with in Child Welfare and Adult Services, but I didn't recognize it in myself, until I stopped drinking. Much of this work is becoming comfortable with and feeling deserving of success, joy, and peace.

✱✱✱

Yesterday something happened that, for the first time in months, made me think about picking up a drink. I did some major box breathing instead. I received a phone call from a man who is organizing our 50th Newark High School Class Reunion. What!? This man must have gotten the wrong person. How could I possibly be old enough to be having a 50th class reunion? When did this happen? Rather than picking up that drink, I took the time to thank God that time has slowed down significantly since I've been alcohol free. I'm thinking I have quite a few reunions left in me.

✱✱✱

A very close and loved family member's drinking has seriously gotten out of control. I misread her admitting that she was drinking too much as a sign that she wanted to talk about it. She knew I had been alcohol free for at least eight months. When I brought up the issue, she reacted with anger (read "fear") and said to me, "Oh, that's right: you are born-again sober." For a New York minute, I let her sarcasm work me over a bit, but I knew she was hurting. I was her, this time last year. Only she can make the decision to put down the glass. And that's okay. I will be here if she ever wants to talk about it. I love her. I wasn't ready until I was. I am, however, sad because I don't think she will talk to me for some time. She is stubborn like me, but she is very astute as I realize I AM born-again sober. And I have learned a painful lesson to let people ask for help instead of offering it.

***

Flashback Friday. Did you ever drink several glasses of wine prior to your significant other coming home from work and, when he came home and asked if you wanted to open a bottle of wine, you smiled, said "yes," and acted like it was your first one?

***

This Easter Sunday marks nine months of sobriety. It hasn't been easy, and I didn't want to do it, but I knew I had to. And here I am. And every single day, I do the work it takes to live life on the other side of alcohol. Happy Easter from this sober chick!

***

I woke up this morning and reflected on Easter without alcohol, an Easter so different on so many levels, including being away from my family because I spent it alone (my choice). I could be present for the day's true meaning. I talked to my dear friend Mary G and told her about my sobriety, took a long walk, baked perfect cinnamon pecan cookies (amazing how cookies turn out when you're not drinking), made COVID masks for my family, and enjoyed a ham dinner delivered by our neighbors.

***

As I finished a new snowflake quilt this week (so, so happy with how it turned out), I realized how much it was an analogy of my new sober life. I largely did my last quilt SUI (sewing under the influence). Overall, it turned out okay if you didn't look too closely at how the corners didn't quite come together. Some squares weren't all that square. I pulled it off, but it wouldn't fool a true quilter. Not too dissimilar to those closest to me who were certainly not fooled about my drinking.

***

Like my many past attempts to quit drinking, I started and stopped writing in many journals. This time, I have written in mine every day since July 12, 2019, and I now see so much value in the practice. It allows me to see my progress, to see just how far I have come, and the words inspire me to keep me moving forward.

***

About 14 years ago, Paul and I did a major kitchen remodel in our old house. The crowning touch was my beautiful, top of the line, dual-temperature-zone wine refrigerator. We took out a small closet in one bedroom to make room for it. I had to have it. Paul thought it was totally ridiculous and unnecessary, but he gave in. It was my pride and joy, until it wasn't. It usually sat empty because of the rate at which I was drinking the contents. We sold that house a few years ago, and unfortunately, my wine habit didn't end with the sale.

***

I no longer feel the need to create drinking events to justify more drinking—Book Club, Rosé Night (dry, of course), Girls Night Out (that was a big one), Margarita Night, Wine Tasting (the one alcohol-related activity I still grieve), Birthdays, Holiday Open Houses (I was the Queen of Halloween), Mondays, Tuesdays … I think you get the point. It's exhausting to even write this entry.

***

I remember starting out drinking Sutter Home rosé because, frankly, it was the only wine I could get down my throat. I eventually "graduated" to a more "sophisticated" palate. Oh, it was so much easier to justify drinking those pricier wines. However, when my drinking escalated, I specialized in sauvignon blanc with twist tops, which were so much more conducive to closet drinking or drinking in the car. Imagine the freedom of not having to carry a corkscrew in your handbag, right? I don't know why I never made the switch to box wines, or wines-in-a-can. I know, however, that I won't waste a single second on trying to solve that mystery.

***

For years, I couldn't get it right. Not. Even. Close. I would string together days, weeks, months, and then slowly (sometimes not so slowly) drink again, often in secret until it became obvious to my family. The outside world was unaware. I was successful at "sweet talking" my husband into letting me drink again, convincing him that I was "okay now" and that this time I could "handle it." That happened over and over and over, until, as you well know, I almost lost everything that meant anything to me.

***

When I would see a younger person getting their life together by removing alcohol from their life, I sometimes regretted that I didn't do it much sooner (even though my drinking became a problem later in life). As much as I would like to turn back the clock, I know there is a reason for everything, and I'm exactly where I need to be. There is great peace in knowing that if something happened to me, I could leave this world knowing that I left it while working to be the best version of myself I could be.

***

Physical books mean something to me again. I rekindled (see what I did there?) my love of bookstores. Ah, the smell of them. I love the visual and tactile feeling of books. I have an emotional connection to them, especially ones that have helped me to understand and sustain my sobriety. I can just feel my progress. *This Naked Mind.* The Sober Diaries. *Drinking: A Love Story. We Are the Luckiest* (so excited to have a signed copy). They feel like family. They feel like hot chocolate. Every book I read about alcohol brings me closer to my truth.

***

Have you ever been told you are "too much"? I have heard this for most of my life from family, friends, teachers, and my husband. "You talk too much." "You're much too sensitive." "You're much too passionate." "You dream too much." "You're being way too emotional about this."

I'm too much for who?

I have always been "too much." My teachers would say, "Peggi, put your hands down." My family would say, "Be more realistic." My husband would say, "When we go in this restaurant/attend this event/sit in these airplane seats, try not to talk to everyone." My husband even made up a signal to let me know I was talking too much. He would brush his hand over his ear. Some of our friends thought this was cute and followed his lead. I sometimes drank to ignore that signal. Well, guess what? I AM all these things, AND I am not "too much" of anything.

I have been told I'm too loud, too crazy, too "seen," too passionate, too friendly, too dramatic, too opinionated. I talk to too many strangers. I have too many ideas, too many dreams. I got straight "A's" but my mom was never happy, because the teachers always checked the box "Needs to practice self-control" as I spoke up in class when no one else would.

I began to doubt myself. I felt this need to dull down my brightness. So, I started drinking at my "too muchness." I drank to hold myself back from being my authentic self. Drinking put me out of alignment with myself. It disconnected me from my core values and I ended up in self-loathing.

> "You're not the same as you were before, he said. You were much more … muchier … you've lost your muchness." [20]
> —Lewis Carroll, Alice's Adventure in Wonderland

> "We, as women still, sadly, live in a world that would sooner see us small, quiet and pleasing than to be 'too much' of anything really. But when we steep and surround ourselves with supports that actually encourage us to be more of who we are, resources that call out and nurture all those disowned and rejected parts of ourselves, when we keep company with those who are not intimidated by our bigness, loudness, boldness, intelligence, ambition, hungers, etc., we give ourselves the nurturing and permission we may need to reclaim our muchness." [21]
> —Annie Wright

My friend Jill's son describes her as being "extra" (so cute). I have owned my past behavior, apologized, made amends. Sobriety is a place where my "too muchness" has a place to shine; where I am appreciated, celebrated, and responded to with "me too's." There is a certain trust, honesty, and transparency in the sober community that keeps us, as my lovely friend Susan Christina says, from shrinking.

Go forth and embrace your muchness.

***

I taught my first virtual class on Friday. I have worked so hard in the last weeks learning the technical part of Zoom and figuring out how to adjust the curriculum from the classroom to the computer screen. It scared me shitless. When I first learned we were going virtual, I cried. I thought my teaching career was over. I felt completely vulnerable. Could I really do this? Yes, I could! Getting sober and putting the work in for that laid the foundation for this major change. I'm sure that if this happened while I was drinking, I wouldn't have even attempted it, or I would have come off like Max Headroom. (Look it up.) There were a few glitches, but overall, a (virtual) success.

***

I am feeling, for the first time in years, that my outside self and my inside self are congruent, in sync, the same, whole. My values of integrity, freedom, justice, growth, curiosity, and humor are aligned. I look each morning in the mirror and love the me I see. Glennon Doyle (haha, can you tell which book I'm reading this week?) puts it perfectly:

"For me sobriety is not just about stopping something … this way of life requires living in integrity: ensuring that my inner self and outer self are integrated. Integrity means having only one self." [22]

Yes, it does.

***

I think we often use the word "failure" when a better word to use would be "pain." Not meeting the expectations you set for yourself can be painful. Getting sober can be painful, because alcohol numbs us from feeling painful things, often for years. I think we should drop the word "failure" from our vocabulary. Instead, we need to ask, "What is this pain trying to teach me and what lies on the other side of it?" Letting pain flow through you is the only way to move closer to your authentic self.

***

Yesterday, when I finished teaching a particularly grueling online class, this Ursula voice I haven't heard in ages popped into my head. "Ah, you deserve a drink now. No one will know. It's just a little drink."

It surprised me the voice was so loud, so strong. At nine months sober, I can honestly say those thoughts have become rare. I answered back: "Sure, I deserve to not remember. I deserve to black out. I deserve to wake up with a hangover and waste my whole fucking day. I deserve to feel like shit about myself. Nope, not today, not today."

***

This morning I was preparing for my virtual class and the internet was down. I freaked out, semi-hysterical, playing the tape over in my head: "What in the hell am I going to do?" Then my sober toolbox kicked in. I did some box breathing, called my co-trainer Luck (That is her actual name), who showed me how to use my phone as a hot spot, and it saved the day. It was another AFGO kind of day.

***

I walk almost every day now and I was thinking how awesomely different it feels from my drinking days when I would walk to temper a hangover. Or I would walk so I could justify coming home and having wine (counteracting all those boozy calories). I would even sometimes walk after I'd been drinking, all the time wondering if my walking partner could smell the wine on my breath.

***

Today is my daughter's 39th birthday. I brought Lindsay her dinner and cake and sat with her and Jason while we watched the grandkids on the trampoline. I haven't seen her or the kids for a couple months because of COVID. As I was sitting there, I couldn't help but replay the damage my drinking caused in our relationship.

In one of her coaching sessions, I asked Laura McKowen about mending my relationship with Lindsay. Her response was: "Relationships are where we feel the most grief. The most beautiful work is making living amends—you are becoming a woman of honor and dignity. It takes time. This is how you will be seen the rest of your living days by your daughter. She may have this work forever, and that's okay. It's not your fault. She is her own animal with her own destiny. We must continually make the decision to forgive ourselves. One thing that's not serving your daughter is holding yourself on the cross. It's not. You can't repair the damage with feeling more shame and more guilt. Give it time, give it grace. You mentioned you didn't know what kind of mother you would find at any given time and that may have been true for your daughter, but it's not true anymore. I wish my mom would engage in even a fraction of this work. I think it's gorgeous and wonderful."

✳✳✳

I wanted to share what my friend Nancy A wrote: "You don't need alcohol to have a good time and there is not a single good time I've had in the last 600 days that would have been IMPROVED by the existence of alcohol … that deeply fulfilling friendships can survive the removal of alcohol and that it's possible to make friends absent the option of going out for a drink, am I right?"

So, in honor of Cinco de Mayo, let's NOT drink together tonight.

✳✳✳

At almost ten months alcohol free, I rarely think about picking up that glass (read: bottle) of wine. Last evening, I walked over to my neighbor's house (socially distancing, of course), with a Gruvi non-alcoholic prosecco in hand. They have been so supportive of my sobriety. These are neighbors I drank and drank and drank with regularly. It's nice to know our friendship survived sobriety. They have told me how proud they are of me. I continue to do the work, not for fear of slipping, but for fear of forgetting just how wonderful, how awesomely messy, my life is now. I never want to go back to the place again where I feel the need to drink to escape it.

***

There are no shortcuts to recovery, no Cliff Notes, no Sober for Dummies, no magic pills. Alcohol is the shortcut. Never underestimate the work it takes to get sober. Get uncomfortable; that is the only place where long-lasting growth happens. Getting sober was harder for me than any college degree I have earned.

***

I realize that there is never a good enough reason to put a drink in my hand. I remember hearing, "Be stronger that your strongest excuse." A friend said to me today: "If I drink, I will lose and I am not down for losing. I want people to know that a drink will never help a situation. It is a rough road to begin with, but the rewards are amazing."

I love that.

***

Three-freaking-hundred alcohol-free days! In numerology, the number 300 represents a sense of infinite potential, optimism, and inspiration for life. These days, my cup does (almost always) feel (at least) half full and I am so proud to end that phrase with "and not with wine."

***

My beautiful-inside-and-out friend and sober sister Kelly B said this yesterday: "I am grateful for how many days I've woken up sober, how many days I've gone to bed sober, how many times I've greeted my children sober without alcohol on my breath, without any guilt in my heart and without any fear of what is to come. It has been an extraordinary year for that and a whole lot of growth."

Amen, sister!

***

On this Mother's Day, two days short of ten months, my priceless gift to my children and grandkids (and, of course, to myself) is that I'm sober. I am grounded and present and authentic and connected. I know emotional sobriety. I am living a bigger life. I am trustworthy and reliable. I am completely humbled by it all. I never thought this was possible. But it is. For anyone who wants something more than they fear it. Happy Mother's Day.

***

I received this text yesterday from Susan: "I am most grateful that 302 days ago you made the decision to love yourself. What a boundless gift to all that know you and to those who will come to know you. For me, I have a dear friend that is authentic, supportive, present, curious, truthful, careful, and safe. Happy Mother's Day, Peggi. Today and always ..."

***

Ten-month soberversary today (after so, so, many day ones). Ten months of growing from the inside out through reading, writing, studying, journaling, meditating, listening, surrendering, crying, Marco-ing, exercising, quilting, feeling, praying, reflecting, connecting, laughing, grieving, paying-it-forward, teaching, supporting, dancing, knowing. I love every person in this community. I am in awe of you. Thank you.

***

One of the "ings" I left off yesterday was "forgiving." Of myself and of others. Last fall, my husband, two of my brothers and their wives were sitting outside after dinner. We were all emotionally drained and on edge from our younger brother's ordeal with heart surgery. My sister-in-law said, "Paul, you must be so proud that Peggi quit drinking." Like I wasn't sitting right there. It felt condescending and quite bitchy to me, and let's just say my reaction made things awkward. My brother Jerry told me that my behavior wasn't cool, and I had an extreme talent for clearing a room in the shortest amount of time. Yep, that's me. Time to follow the advice of the chick from Frozen and let it go. Holding grudges serves no purpose in my new life. Sis, I am sorry from the bottom of my heart. I love you dearly.

***

My daughter had me over for dinner on Mother's Day, and she was even quieter than her usual quiet self. My shame/guilt voice started talking to me: "She hasn't forgiven you. She will never forgive you." I said: "Stop, Peggi, she's probably just tired, she was at a brunch all day with mimosas flowing, she's teaching kindergarteners online and homeschooling two eight-year-old twins. She probably feels comfortable enough around you to just be herself. It's not about you."

This is what emotional sobriety looks like.

***

I am loving James Clear's book *Atomic Habits*. He talks about implementation intentions.

> "Being specific about what you want and how you will achieve it helps you to say NO to things that derail progress, distract you, and pull you off course." [23]

I call this planning. Always being prepared. You cannot be vague about your intention to be alcohol free. You must have a plan. You must do the work. Every. Damn. Day.

***

My director from the university I work for called me today. Nothing good can come from a call at 3:00 pm on a Friday, right? My body immediately filled with cortisol. She wanted to discuss my being overheard talking about a difficult student. (I was unaware there was anyone else on the Zoom call; however, I had no business discussing this person in the first place.) The intense pain from the shame I felt was on par with my last drinking incident in July. My heart hurt. My director was so compassionate. She said, "I know who you are. I adore you. Please know that I know it was a one-time thing." I owned it, gave myself compassion, knowing this experience will make me a better human. I'm just so grateful alcohol didn't fit into the equation.

***

I haven't read one post since I started this journey on July 12, 2019, of someone posting any of the following: "I drank last night, and it was amazing!" "I am so glad I drank at that wedding yesterday, made a complete ass out of myself and lost my wallet." "I am so proud that I passed out in front of my grandchildren." "I am so proud that I can't remember a fucking thing about last night."

However, I do read multiple posts about how great it is to wake up in the morning after a good night's sleep and being able to remember everything about the night before.

***

Am I a way better mother, wife, friend, teacher, listener, writer now that I am alcohol free? No doubt. Do I miss (will I miss) sipping a chilled glass of crisp sauvignon blanc with a friend or enjoying a mai tai with the hubs from Mama's Fish House or the Monkeypod Kitchen on Maui? Absolutely! Both things are true, and that's okay.

***

A Facebook memory reminded me that this time last year, Paul and I were traveling to Mallorca, Spain, for my husband's cycling tour. I remember hating the world because, once again, I wasn't drinking because of a blackout incident that happened in early March in front of my stepdaughter, followed by threats of cancelling the trip altogether. How could I possibly have any fun without drinking? After a stressful baggage and passport debacle in Barcelona, I talked Paul into having a drink and, sadly, that was all it took to go down the rabbit hole again. Two months later, I found Sober Sis.

***

My Marco sister Ellen texted a picture of us that was taken at the Sober Sis retreat in October 2019. I was close to 100 days alcohol free. I remember the day we took it and how awful I thought I looked in it. I have never liked pictures of myself, and I have very few of them. When I looked at it this time, I had the opposite reaction. I thought it was a flattering picture of both of us. What was different? I have clearly been changing on the inside.

***

I have officially dropped these words from my vocabulary: always, never, and forever. They can leave us feeling deprived or feeling like we are missing out. Instead, I think in terms of now. I am not going to drink NOW. This mindset has served me well for 315 days and counting.

***

On my walk this morning, I came upon a neighbor who introduced himself to me as if he hadn't met me before. He didn't remember that less than a year ago, he and his wife invited us in to see his remodel and to share a cocktail (or two) at his new custom-built bar. It was obvious then that these weren't his first drinks of the evening. I wonder how many times I have introduced myself to someone again, as if for the first time?

***

Occasionally, I mindlessly compare my past addiction to others'. I listened to a man who spoke about how he had to scrape his face off rock bottom several times before he got sober. I thought to myself: I was never THAT bad. OMG, who was I kidding? Almost losing my daughter, grandkids, and my marriage wasn't rock bottom enough for me? It's crazy how our mind works sometimes, and how much wasted time we spend rationalizing our behavior. It's not how much we drink, but what happens to you when you drink.

***

I woke up this morning with thoughts of my alcohol-free "firsts": Halloween, Thanksgiving, Christmas, New Year's Eve/Day, Super Bowl, Valentine's Day, Easter, Mother's Day, My Birthday, Memorial Weekend. Just one more to go before I hit a year: July 4. How fitting is that? It hasn't been easy, but I'm at peace and comfortable in my skin. I don't have to be sober. I get to be.

***

I give myself permission to be sad now. This is a monumental shift for me.

"Your sadness is trying to reach you and carry away things no longer meant for you; if you're sad, BE sad; sadness [can be] a beautiful flowing emotion." [24]—Laura McKowen

81

We should not be afraid of sadness, as it's simply not possible to feel good all of the time. My ultimate goal is not to think in terms of happy and sad; but rather, to think in terms of simply being at peace, being whole. It may be comforting to know that the only people who are always free of sadness are dead ones.

Australian sociologist Hugh McKay expresses this concept perfectly:

"I had an amazing conversation last night with a person who I really love. We talked about how often we see people shy away from 'negative' emotions, and how it's so much easier to let them go when we allow ourselves to experience them. I actually attack the concept of happiness. The idea that—I don't mind people being happy—but the idea that everything we do is part of the pursuit of happiness seems to me a really dangerous idea and has led to a contemporary disease in Western society, which is fear of sadness. It's a really odd thing that we're now seeing people saying 'write down three things that made you happy today before you go to sleep' and 'cheer up' and 'happiness is our birthright' and so on. We're kind of teaching our kids that happiness is the default position. It's rubbish. Wholeness is what we ought to be striving for and part of that is sadness, disappointment, frustration, failure; all of those things which make us who we are. Happiness and victory and fulfillment are nice little things that also happen to us, but they don't teach us much. Everyone says we grow through pain and then as soon as they experience pain they say, 'Quick! Move on! Cheer up!' I'd like just for a year to have a moratorium on the word 'happiness' and to replace it with the word 'wholeness.' Ask yourself, 'Is this contributing to my wholeness?' and if you're having a bad day, it is." [25]

THIS SIDE OF ALCOHOL

***

I came across my favorite quote by Tony Robbins this morning. (If you know him, imagine Tony being Tony and practically yelling this.)

> "If you're going to blame people for all the shit, you better blame them for all the good too. If you're going to give them credit for everything that's fucked up, then you have to give them credit for everything that's great. I'm not asking you to stop blaming. I'm saying, blame elegantly, blame intelligently, blame effectively, blame at the level of your soul, not the level of your fucking head." [26]

I needed this quote in the worst way today. I would love to say it to a couple of family members who have blamed me and cut me out of their lives without considering all the good I have done. Family members who have looked at, listened to, only one side of the story. I know all of my messes and the successes are the reason I am "here." And "here" is an excellent place to be.

***

I'm not gonna lie. Sometimes sobriety has been harder than shit for me. Some days just getting up every morning and going to bed sober is all I can do. But you know what's harder than becoming alcohol free? Thinking about it and staying in the same miserable (and I mean miserable) place. Day after day. Nothing creates more inner conflict than wanting to change and doing nothing about it. I had a friend say to me, "A year from now you'll wish you would have started today."

So, I did. I started the Sober Sis reset two weeks early. I haven't looked back.

***

I let go of regrets about not starting on my alcohol-free journey sooner. I am exactly where I need to be and doing exactly what I am supposed to be doing right now—writing, learning, connecting, healing. I wonder how many messages I missed while my mind was altered, too numbed out with alcohol to receive them. Thank God for this "do over." Universe, I promise I won't let you down. I am here now. I plan to stick around.

***

When I stopped drinking almost eleven months ago, I believed 100% that I would completely stop having or being fun. I hated everyone and everything. I couldn't imagine living alcohol free. But guess what? I'm sober and I'm not bored or boring (my unbiased observation). I am fun and funny (again, unbiased). I experience SFBL (spontaneous full body laughter) regularly. Sobriety has truly been the best adventure of my life.

***

I woke up yesterday mad at the entire world for no apparent reason. (I have learned to appreciate these unpredictable AF mood swings.) Before sobriety, I'd have wallowed in my "madness" for days. But I've learned that nothing gets me out of my own way faster than being of service to others. Paying it forward is part of recovery. Helping others gets you out of your head spiral. Writing encouraging and supportive posts to others in recovery, making phone calls, sending private messages, are all small things you can do that connect you to humanity.

"For it is in the giving that we receive." [27] —St. Francis of Assisi

***

I'm sure I couldn't deal with what's happening in our country, in my state, in my city, and in my neighborhood if I were still drinking. COVID, more fires, civil unrest. Completely unprecedented times. How do you feel stable in a world that is inherently not? I don't know how to find peace, seek solutions, without sobriety. My life doesn't work without it.

***

Only in sobriety would I ever have taken on five granddaughters for a three-day weekend. There was putting, walking, board/card gaming, hot tubbing, storytelling, crafting, barbequing, charcuterie trays, s'mores, G-pa's famous waffles, watching G-ma's favorite movies with popcorn of course—Edward Scissorhands, Never-

84

Ending Story, The Labyrinth, Princess Bride. I loved the craziness of being together.

***

I show up! Every day. For myself and for others. I don't cancel shit. I follow through. I call people back. I get stuff done. I mark off things on my list. I am of service to others. That was almost always true for my job and colleagues, but alcohol would often make it untrue for my family and friends. Not anymore.

"My thing is alcohol, but I am not drinking it." [28]
—Laura McKowen

***

Whenever a glass of wine sounds amazing, like after teaching a Zoom class from hell on Tuesday (the hell wasn't because of the students, it was all Zoom), I picture that morning in July when I almost lost everything I love. I get choked up every damn time I write, talk, or think about that day. Still. No glass of wine, nor its ten minutes of a dopamine rush, is worth losing my family.

***

In my work as a direct practice social worker, I was mindful not to use demeaning words to describe parents struggling with addiction. Lazy. Selfish. Crazy. How-can-they-love-drugs/alcohol-more-than-their-kids? Weak. Mental. And then I was the receiver of those same words from my husband. In all fairness, after he read *This Naked Mind* and *Alcohol Explained*, he understood the impact of those words. I wonder, though, whether had he not used those words and instead had tried to love me through it, my drinking might not have gone underground (and into my closet). That's when things spiraled out of control for me. Yes, there is still a lot to forgive on both sides.

***

Saying "no" to alcohol is making it possible for me to say "yes" to so many things—things I was too numbed out for or too tired to do when I was drinking. I have opportunities to get to know people better. I can actually listen now. I notice things. I can make a phone call, make someone's day, walk a little further, make a new sober friend, read another chapter, stop and smell a rose (for real!). I am saying "yes" to myself more every day. I have become the CEO of my own life.

***

Last night I had dinner with a new sober friend, Julie, who was driving through the 916 on the way home from work. She called up at the last minute to see if I was available. This time last year, I probably would have declined because, sadly, I eliminated anything from my life that wasn't work-related, or post-work wine-related. We enjoyed a beautiful dinner, conversation, and sunset at Rio City Café on the Sacramento River. Outdoor dining had just opened after four months of COVID-related shutdowns. It was an evening of fun and laughter, with only a tinge of jealousy for the man sitting at the next table with his glass of white wine.

***

As I approach my one-year anniversary, my mind has been flooded with memories of all the dumb-ass, dangerous, and brainless things I did that I would never have dreamed of doing had I been sober. This is a common effect that many of my sober friends experienced as they approached their own anniversaries. Ugh, all the mental and physical scars. How did I ever think what I was doing was normal? I'm sure that these thoughts are messages from God, who is telling me: "If you are considering you might drink again, let's recap why that wouldn't be a wise decision."

***

The problem with using alcohol to numb out my pain was that I couldn't feel my joy either.

***

Today, I am 11 months sober. I am full of hope. Hope differs completely from wanting. I wanted to stop drinking for at least five years, but after so many day ones I had lost hope. I just couldn't see how life could be better without drinking until I found Jenn (or did she find me?) and the Sober Sis community, where I went from feeling hopeless to hopeful about the future. From I will never be able to do this to I am most definitely doing this.

THIS SIDE OF ALCOHOL

***

I was listening to Jenn Elizabeth's (*Shape of a Woman*), who said:

> "Stay [in recovery] for whatever reason you are here.
> Your reason to stay will change in the end." [29]

I started this journey because I was so close to losing my relationship with my daughter and grandkids, and for sure, I was about to lose my marriage. I stayed because my life is infinitely better. I stayed because I am one version of myself. I stayed because my life has purpose.

***

Breathing has become an essential sobriety tool. Simple box breathing—breathe in, hold for 4, breathe out, hold for 4. It calms my central nervous system like no other technique. I breathe before I teach a class, when I need to be present, before I feel like totally unloading on my husband, when the clerks at the store would rather talk about their dates last Saturday night than wait on me, before I flip off the driver who just cut me off on the freeway, before I let something that someone said to me hurt my feelings, before I fall asleep. Jenn Kautsch posted that "breathe" is her word for 2020. "It came to me before the craziness of this year. Just like you said. Breathe in, breathe out, it is life."

***

I was looking to see when my next cardiologist appointment was and I came across this on my health record: alcohol use disorder, full remission. I first went to see a cardiologist after my brother's massive heart attack last fall. (Our father died at 47 from a widow maker, and our older brother had a heart attack at 57, so obviously I had reason to worry about my own heart health.) I remember feeling so proud at the time that I was honest with her about my drinking history. Not sure why she felt the need to write that in my permanent record. And not sure why I felt so betrayed by it. Being honest was clearly important to my health and to accurately plan my future heart care, but "alcohol use disorder"? Seeing it in black and white, "on the record," just plain hurt.

***

I used to brag that I was the kind of person who could fit in anywhere and with anyone, that I could be comfortable around both drug dealers and royalty. A chameleon. A shape shifter. With alcohol, there were so many versions of myself, I basically didn't know who I was. In sobriety, I am one version of myself. I get to be me, albeit a life of extensive work in progress: Take it or leave it. I gotta be me. Or as Popeye wisely exclaims: "I yam what I yam."

***

As I move nearer to that one-year milestone of sobriety, so many thoughts and feelings are bubbling up for me. I think about all the times I have stopped drinking over the past five years, some lasting only a few hours, some a few days, some a few weeks, and others turning into months. Sometimes I said I stopped drinking, but I was lying. I cannot start over again. Like so many others, I don't have another sobriety in me.

***

When I write these posts, I am often scared shitless, far out of my comfort zone. The more real and raw, the more vulnerable I feel. Are my words too much, too trivial, too shocking, too personal, too triggering, too shallow? I do it anyway because not living my truth is far scarier than putting myself out there every day. I write in heart-felt hope that my courage will inspire some of you to face your own fears about drinking.

***

Teaching social work has turned me into such a brain science geek. Getting sober has increased the geek. When we quit drinking, our brains heal from the inside out. Going alcohol free heals our brain in five ways: there is regeneration of the frontal lobe where decision making and impulse control happen; dopamine levels normalize; motivation increases; serotonin production increases; and your brain builds new connections and neuropathways that promote emotional sobriety. I marvel at how we can flood our brains

88

with ethanol, and yet when we stop, our brains are resilient enough to reverse the abuse and heal.

***

This is what I know at day 347. You must do the work, period. There is absolutely no judgment in this. I wasn't ready to do the work until I was. Staying alcohol free is my number one job. It comes before my family, my friends, my career. I don't have any of these blessings without sobriety. If that means not attending that party, that gathering, that family event, I don't. Without guilt. This time is about ME. I do the work every single day. The life I want literally depends on it.

***

When I took my last drink on July 11, 2019, I couldn't imagine ever having fun again. I was so conditioned to believe that alcohol was such a central component of my life, I just knew that not drinking would make me a very boring person. How could there possibly be life after sauvignon blanc? Slowly I found myself (my real self) seeing and feeling what the world had to offer sans alcohol. I wasn't good at it at first. Alcohol doesn't make us interesting. That's up to us. I had to practice. I had to make myself do things (or not do things) that weren't really me.

***

I was talking yesterday morning with one of my sober friends, Alice, and we both admitted to hearing "those" voices as we neared that one-year milestone. "Yay, you made it to a year. Let's celebrate with a little Brut." "Just a little sip … what harm could it do?" "You've already shown you can use self-control." "Everyone is still drinking and you're not." The struggle is real. The voices are loud, but we are louder.

***

In the past, my family made fun of me because I would rarely (I mean rarely) leave the house without doing my hair and makeup, even when I went camping or just out walking. I was carrying so much shame on the inside, that I thought I could fool people by trying to look good on the outside. Now, I often go out "au naturel", adding one more freedom that comes with being AF.

***

I listen to music every day—when I get ready in the morning, on my daily walks, and on long drives. I often sing along, loudly, and totally off key (thanks, Mom). I dance in my kitchen. My current favorites are "*You Go Down Smooth*" (Lake Street Dive), "*I Love Me*" (Meghan Trainor), "*Yes, We Can Can*" (The Pointer Sisters), "*Happy*" (Pharrell Williams), "*7 Years*" (Lukas Graham), and "*I'm Still Standing*" (Elton John, who has been sober for 30 years).

***

I have spent so much of this first year taking the time to understand my past hurts. We can heal traumatic memories with time, but only if you do the work necessary to allow them to flow through you. In the beginning, we only see the tip of the iceberg, those things that everyone sees on the outside. As we dig deeper, we lower the waterline and uncover the underlying reasons for our behavior. Some painful memories fade into lessons learned, some become priceless gifts, and some are ones I never want to forget.

I tended to compare my hurts and traumas to other's and mine seemed relatively small. My daughter's death was tragic, I told myself, but it wasn't like losing an older child. I never experienced what experts term "Big T" traumas. Mine all qualified as "Little t" traumas: conflict with family members, divorce, sudden relocation, working with trauma survivors, conflict at work, and one I have suffered from for most of my life but have never talked about to anyone.

Puberty for me came late in my 15th year. Before that happened, I was flat-chested, 5'8", and weighed 120 pounds. I was proud of my post-puberty body. I have one picture of me in my bikini standing in front of my dad's ski boat at Lake Berryessa. A little over a year later, I was pregnant. Having a child at 17 left my body covered in stretch marks because I wasn't done growing yet. When my baby died, those stretch marks and less-than-perky boobs became a symbol of deep shame. Who would ever want me? I was damaged goods. I continued to feel that way throughout every romantic relationship. I have always been self-conscious about my body.

It's so crazy that now I have done the work, I am more than okay with those stretch marks. I am proud of this 68-year-old body.

***

I went to the eye doctor yesterday without the usual dread and anxiety I used to feel when I was drinking: Could he smell the alcohol on my breath from the night before? Would he comment on my bloodshot eyes? Would he notice my shaking hands? Would my prescription even be accurate? Completely sober, it is still so weirdly awkward being eye to eye with a person you aren't intimate with, right? And, while I have you, I'd like to take this opportunity for an educational moment for all of us: drinking can contribute to increased age-related macular degeneration, increased cataract formation, dry eye, and blurred vision.

***

Twenty years ago, I drove a mother on my child welfare caseload to rehab. Her hands were shaking so badly, I had to fill out the admission paperwork. She couldn't even sign her name. I had been working with this mom for a couple years, and I remember being so happy she finally agreed to enter a program. I remember thinking, "How could she choose alcohol over her three beautiful children?" I was so dumb. So ignorant. She ended up dying from cirrhosis of the liver ten years later.

Little did I know that alcohol would wreak havoc in my own life, and I would look down to see my own hands shaking. Rest in peace, dear R. I will take it from here.

***

Sobriety has taught me the art of purposefully taking a pause, waiting a few seconds before speaking, a gift born from mindfulness. I have come to look at taking a pause as a circuit breaker. I find I am a much nicer person to my husband: He leaves the burner on; I just turn it off. He leaves the garage door open all night; I close it. Toilet seat up? Technically unforgivable, but I put it down (most of the time, unless it's dark and I fall in and then all bets are off). I am not constantly pointing out the things he does or says that irritate me, except, of course, when he doesn't replace the toilet paper. That IS unforgivable. My friend Susan B said that being sober-minded allows her to use her "defense mechanism less" and helps her to be less offended by silly things. Susan speaks the truth.

***

I came across this Anne Lamott quote today. Her words describe exactly how I felt when I found Sober Sis and The Luckiest Club. This is me. This is us.

> "So, I showed up … there were all of these women who had what I had, who'd thought what I thought, who'd done what I'd done, who betrayed their families and deepest values, who sat with me that day and said, Guess what? Me too! I have that too. Let me get you a glass of water. Those are the words of salvation. Guess what? Me too."[30]

I have never felt more at home, more understood, more accepted by humans in my entire life.

***

Teaching social work for the last six years has been my absolute dream job. For five of those years, I was carrying a dark secret. I was teaching by day and breaking my family's heart by night. I was excelling in my career in every way, and I was struggling with my relationship with wine. There were significant periods of time where I didn't drink, followed by failed attempts at moderation. I felt like a complete fraud. Not now. Ahh, freedom. This is the best Fourth of July I have had in years. Happy Fourth, everyone!

***

The hubs asked me this yesterday: "Aren't you close to being done with all the meetings, courses, work you are doing? I mean, it's almost been a year, right?"

Because I feel I have single-handedly discovered the secret of life, my first thought was to put up a vigorous defense. I took a big breath and calmly answered: "No, I am not done. I will most likely never be done. It has become my life's purpose." And I added this with a slight, adoring grin: "I couldn't have done this without your support." He smiled and said, "Okay."

***

I am in awe of our yard this year. The plants and flowers appear to be on steroids. Paul is the master gardener, but I find myself spending more time watering, dead-heading the flowers, and pulling weeds. All of this is so much more enjoyable without a hangover. It's the same with the work of sobriety. When it comes to the workings of the heart and mind, we also have to water, dead-head, and pull those weeds. Whatever you water grows.

***

Today, July 8, is my husband's birthday, marking the last milestone before reaching one year without alcohol. This means that I can look back on every holiday and birthday since July 11, 2019, without shame, without regret, without self-hatred. It has been far from easy. I chose to spend many of them by myself. It has been a peaceful year. Happy birthday, Paul.

***

One of the biggest gifts of this crazy sober COVID year has been the love, the cheerleading, the unconditional support of my recovery communities. I love you. I got you. I am rooting for you. My husband cannot fathom how I could make such deep friendships and connections with women, so many of you I have not (yet) met in person. "How can you be close to people you have only met online?" He has no clue. Nor do I expect him to. Y'all know more about my life than most of my other friends and family. We share our pain, joy, struggles, and milestones with equal enthusiasm. I hear you. I see you. All of you have been foundational in changing the trajectory of my life. Lifelong friendships have formed and will continue to grow. Geez, my eyes are doing that leaking thing again. Saying I am grateful just doesn't seem to be enough.

***

A couple of days ago, a very heavy Amazon package arrived on my porch. I opened it and there were five bags of birdseed. I panicked. Memories of my ordering-on-Amazon-under-the-influence days came flooding back—days where I had to pretend I knew what was in the damn box, when I had no clue. I couldn't for the life of me remember ordering birdseed. Of course, I knew I didn't drink, but I was worried my memory might be slipping. My husband was worried, too. I ran to the computer—no birdseed order, thank God. Checked the name on the box and yep, it was my name. Then I realized I'd had a conversation with my good friend Alice about all the beautiful birds in our yard this year and realized she must have sent it to me in advance of my soberversary. I love you so much, Alice, but you scared the shit out of me. This moment brought to you by the Universe, with another reminder of why I never want to go back there.

***

A colleague and I were at a social work training in San Diego a few months ago and I saw this quote printed on the restroom mirror: "You are the best thing that can happen to anyone."

I took a selfie. I am a believer. I lived through events this year that I never thought I could do sober. I can sit with cravings and don't need to act on them. I have become very good at saying "no" and/or leaving early when I feel uncomfortable. I trust myself. I have self-compassion. I talk to myself the way I would talk to my children or to a friend. I am confident I will not return to the person I wasn't. I'm not afraid to take on new things. I am also a realist. I cannot sing, draw, or play an instrument. I am banned from playing Pictionary in my family. Everything I draw looks like a cat. When my kids were young, they begged me not to practice playing the saxophone because I was single-handedly changing the migration patterns of geese. Rude.

I may not be able to sing, draw, or play an instrument, but I have always been a hell of a choreographer. I am an excellent connector. Being sober has allowed me to enhance those gifts and apply them every day.

Chapter Six

Transformation
(The second year – Unbroken)

"Open the door to possibilities. Stop drinking and start loving yourself." *–Louise Atthey*

Today is July 12, 2020. It's the first anniversary of my last day one (366 days in a leap year).

I gave a first-time-grandma baby shower for a friend of 34 years. We were setting up for the party and I shared with her that it coincided with my being alcohol free for a year. She responded, "I didn't realize you had such a problem." Ugh.

Then later, in front of all the guests, she shared about a time where she confronted me about my lying about how much I had to drink one evening at our cabin. "Yep," I answered. "People who have an unhealthy relationship with alcohol have a tendency to lie about their drinking." [Ed. note: Stories like this used to be funny: recounting how I made an ass out of myself. I used to welcome them. I never realized how painful they would become.]

And then I remembered how this friend was there for me whenever, wherever I needed her. We were Thelma and Louise. I realized that none of her words were coming from a critical place. My sobriety sensitivity runs deep.

Later that evening, my friend Susan surprised me with her homemade Meyers lemon cupcakes spelled out to say "AF." I ate every single one. No guilt. No shame.

***

My initial year of sobriety was more about documenting my recovery and holding myself accountable—observations, really, of people, places, and feelings along my sobriety path. Some of it was overwhelming, but my first year went by surprisingly fast. That wasn't something I'd expected.

In year two, I feel like I have a new brain and I feel 15 years younger.

I'm pretty sure I'm having more fun than my kids and as much fun as my grandkids.

The further I walk down the AF path, the more I move towards the alignment of my external and internal worlds. I don't want to jinx anything, but this year feels more like sobriety has become second nature to me. I'm thinking in sober. I'm busy teaching, writing, taking part in the recovery community. Yet my life feels so much simpler and peaceful.

As a social worker, I see that transformational change is becoming a new focus in child welfare practice in California. The goal of this practice is to help parents and caretakers make long-lasting behavior changes in their lives that will keep their children safe long after child welfare steps out of the picture. I couldn't help but see the parallel in my own transformation of physical and emotional sobriety.

Transformational thinking includes positive shifts in habits and lifestyle. It's not merely stopping a harmful behavior like drinking; it's choosing to replace that behavior with a healthy one. It's growth-oriented thinking that is necessary for attempting any goal or change in one's life. Transformational change requires the practice of self-awareness and honesty, looking at the factors and experiences that contributed to our behavior. This explains my many long periods of sobriety and the repetitive returning to drinking. I never did the actual work it took to make long-lasting changes that go far beyond white knuckling. Until now.

Transformational change requires that we face the most brutal facts about ourselves, facts that may not be our fault, but facts just the same—and for me, at times, that has been painful. Drinking had become the brilliant cover for my pain. Father Richard Rohr explains this beautifully:

"If we do not transform our pain, we will most assuredly transmit it—usually to those closest to us; our family, our neighbors, our co-workers, and invariably, the most vulnerable, our children." [31] I had become a transmission expert. Until I wasn't.

> I know in the deepest parts of me that "recovery isn't just about not drinking—it's about learning how to thrive so much that drinking becomes unappealing" [32]—*Liv's Recovery Kitchen.*

***

One of my sober superpowers (are you keeping count?) has been my vision board—you know, a collage of your future self, the life you want to live. I'm a total believer. Thank you, Staci Danford and The Grateful Brain. I accomplished four of five of my first board visions: being sober for 366 leap-year days, posting every day on the Sober Sis Facebook page, making my snowflake quilt, and being a presenter at a national coaching conference (virtually, of course, but I'll take it). The only thing I didn't get to do was learn to drive a Can Am Spyder motorcycle with my friend Jan, and that was only because of COVID. That will have to carry over to my next vision board, which includes learning to golf (I mean, I live on a damn golf course), finishing and publishing my book, creating a podcast, going public with my sobriety, and creating my own Facebook and web page. I have done vision boards with my eight-year-old twin granddaughters, and they are begging to do another. What if YOUR vision board came true?

***

One of the biggest gifts of sobriety has been to have those "feel-good" emotions back. Because, when you numb out with alcohol, you numb out the good stuff, too. One of those emotions is "awe," a feeling of reverential respect mixed with wonder. I have my awe back. And it doesn't have to be huge, like standing on a bridge over Niagara Falls or witnessing that perfect Maui sunset. Every day when I take a walk, Nature is a constant "awe-maker" for me. And if you forget what awe feels like, just take a three-year-old on your next walk and, guaranteed, she or he will point out everything wonderful about the world that you would otherwise walk past.

***

I love this saying: "Friendship is so weird … you just pick a human you've met and you're like 'yep, I like this one' and you just do stuff with them." I am learning I'm not afraid to reach out to people who resonate with me. I reach out every day with my posts, and many of you have reached out to me in return. That has been a gift beyond measure. The connections and the friendships have become foundational pieces in my sober-minded life puzzle. I am continuously finding new friends who align with my new values (well, values I have had all along but had been violating with booze). Laura McKowen says it perfectly: "One stranger who understands your experience exactly will do for you what hundreds of close friends and family who don't understand cannot." Don't be afraid to reach out. Not one of us can do this thing alone. I don't even want to try.

***

Did you know that the average drinking person spends two years of their life hungover? Two. Whole. Fucking. Years. Alicia Gilbert puts it this way:

> "I used to wonder how some people found the time and energy to have so much going on in their lives. It turns out that not getting trashed several times a week helps." [33]

Ditto. I have been so hungover that just seeing the sun hurt. I have memories of being so sick post-drinking, I felt like I had eaten an entire cat. (Sorry, cat lovers.) I experienced a stage five hangover where there couldn't possibly have been one single drop of moisture left in my entire body. Sitting with my head on a table at a restaurant where no one was permitted to utter a single word to me because it made my head hurt even more, if that were possible. And the coup de grâce was waking up after consuming two entire bottles of wine at dinner the night before and having to sit and listen to the Marine Corps band play loudly in the grand ballroom at a conference on child maltreatment in San Diego. I had to go back (practically crawl) to my hotel room. I threw up for hours. I was sick for days. Good times.

***

One of the dumbest and most wasteful things I did was lie to my psychologist about my drinking. The only reason I made an appointment with her in the first place was because my husband was furious about my drinking and its impact on our marriage and children. And, right up to the incident that brought me into recovery, I presented myself as a moderate drinker. "I drink a couple glasses of wine while fixing dinner." What made me lie in a confidential, protective environment of a therapy room? Guilt. Shame. And a shitload of it. I was "managing my image," wasting over $2,000, talking about everything but the reason for which I came to get help.

This sober-minded community helped me to come completely clean with her because I realized there were so many of us dealing with the same issue. I cannot tell you how important teaming up with my psychologist has been to my sobriety. I come prepared for each session with recent information, challenges and "aha" moments to discuss. And I love that I have become a resource of information for her to pass on to other clients who are struggling with alcohol.

***

At a little over a year without alcohol, things are running smoothly in our house. There are still many things to work on, of course, especially my relationship with my stepdaughters, but overall, I have very little to complain about. Yesterday, I was reflecting on those first few months of going alcohol free. On one hand, I was relieved. The gig was up. I had dreamed of a life other than the one I had been living. On the other hand, almost everything my husband did irritated the shit out of me! For real! His words often felt like fingernails on a chalkboard. If he left a cupboard door open or replaced the toilet paper roll with the paper rolling out the bottom, I would become irate. He couldn't do anything right. He was hurt; I was hurt. I was one raw nerve, and he was consistently standing on it. I wonder if he ever thought I should start drinking again. The point is, if you are new to sobriety and feeling like this, it is 100% normal and it does go away. Except the toilet paper. That is unacceptable. Always.

***

I planned on posting something entirely different today, but I'm learning to listen to that voice inside my head and my heart that says, "No, Peggi. This is what you need to write about today." I just had to give a shout-out to the recovery communities I am involved with: Sober Sis, We Are the Luckiest, and Soberish. The support I get from the members often brings me literally to my knees. Without it, I honestly don't know where I would be. I certainly wouldn't be here, posting daily to thousands of people who are loving, who accept each other no matter where they are on their sober-minded path, consistently inspire and cheer each other on, transcending all ages (one of my favorit-est parts!). Our community is safe, provides accountability, and expands the horizons for every one of us, no matter where we are on the sober-minded continuum. Every single day. Does anyone remember the song from Jackie DeShannon? Maybe only those of us over 60.

"What the world needs now, is love, sweet love. It's the only thing that's there's just too little of." [34]

Maybe the rest of the world could take a lesson from us sober folks.

***

My sister-in-law came over yesterday to use our internet to teach her class. She is a nurse practitioner. I haven't seen her in over a year.

She said I looked great and asked what I've been doing. I took a chance and told her I stopped drinking over a year ago. The first thing she asked me was, "Are you going to AA?" I said, "No. I joined several recovery communities, took courses, read a shitload of books, and I'm writing a book of my own." She told me that, basically, all people who struggle with drinking are alcoholics. I told her I hate labels of any kind and that the percentage of people physically addicted to alcohol is relatively small; most people who struggle with drinking are psychologically dependent. Saying that to her didn't prevent the residual shame filling my body with cortisol. Damn it. So, I put my big girl panties on and told her I refuse to accept "alcoholic" as my identity and said I was going to go for a walk.

Having an education doesn't mean understanding what alcohol dependence is and isn't. That kind of attitude has the potential to push it underground, as it did to me. It's difficult to talk about addiction when you feel you are being judged. As Holly Whitaker said:

> "… instead of looking at how insane it is to consume the amounts of alcohol we do in this country at any level, we've instead systematically labeled anyone who can't hang in that insanity as having the problem." [35]

Thank you, Holly. My sentiments exactly.

***

I grew up in a chaotic family environment, always expecting the other shoe to drop at any minute. If we were on a great family trip, a huge fight would break out between my parents. One time my parents took me and my cousin to Monterey. We had the best day on the beach and at the Monterey Bay Cannery. When we got back in the car, my mother accidentally scraped the bottom of the car door on the curb. Dad went ballistic, yelling at her: "Shit, Margaret!" (Imagine the word "shit" to have at least ten syllables.) My mother got out of the car and wouldn't get back in. I begged and begged her to get back in the car. My parents' behavior completely mortified me in front of my cousin, whose parents never so much as raised their voices at each other. My dad drove away without my mother. My cousin and I cried all the way home. I cried all night. My mother didn't come home until the next day. I found out later she went to a movie and took the bus home. She was so proud of herself. I hated her. I hated them both.

This view of my world carried over into adulthood. Into my relationships. Into my marriage. Into my parenting. I couldn't shake the belief that whenever things were going well, the bottom would fall out—and if it didn't, I would make sure to fuck things up. Addressing this addiction to chaos is central in the work I am doing to heal.

***

With all the deep work I have done and continue to do, I can truthfully say I have forgiven myself for all the grief I caused my family with my drinking. I do find that I sometimes keep my husband at a distance. This is something I am committed to working on in this year two of sobriety. Some of my words may sound harsh, but I need to get them on paper so that I can get rid of them because the longer I hold on, the more they damage and create distance in our relationship:

> Paul:
>
> When you nagged, pressured, and threatened me to stop, I fell further into self-loathing, and I ended up drinking more just to be around you. Belittling me made me feel worthless. Calling me crazy, mental, having a weak character and selfish helped to push my drinking into the closet (literally) and I turned into the biggest liar on the planet.
>
> Pretty much every time you threatened to leave me or left (and you had every reason to), I would numb myself by drinking to not feel the pain. In all fairness to you, I don't remember ever really asking for your help. It was easier to blame you than look in the mirror.

You told your adult daughters many personal things about our marriage (just my secrets, not yours) that you had absolutely no business sharing and now, my relationship with them seems forever fractured. Did you ever think about how you might have contributed to my drinking? Did you ever consider that loving me through this might have produced a different outcome?

I am not minimizing the hell my drinking put you through. I have forgiven myself. I need to forgive you. Our marriage depends on it. I know you are trying very hard now. I needed to get this off my chest so that I can move forward.

***

I was looking back at texts between Lindsay and me about this time last year and came across a text where she sent me a list of outpatient rehabs. Ouch! At that time, she was as convinced as her stepsisters that Sober Sis wasn't enough to address my drinking. The feelings of shame and heart pain came flooding back like it was yesterday. Then I said, "Stop, Peggi." I took out my journals and read some of the things that have happened with our relationship since that time. I remember wanting to isolate from her and the kids because I literally hated myself. I thought I had made the full transition of turning into my mother.

But I didn't isolate. I did the opposite. I read an entry where I had talked to Cindy in my Marco group, who gave me so much love and encouragement that I just put myself out there. I embraced every chance to spend time with Lindsay and the kids. We went on walks, spent time at the cabin, took the grandkids for weekends, and went with them to Club Center to have dinner and watch the kids swim. ("Hey, Grandma, watch me!") I shared and continue to share every sober milestone with Lindsay and sent her the magazine where I wrote a brief article on "Rethinking Drinking."

A lot can change in a year.

***

When I was hired by a local university to teach social work, a complete dream job, you might have thought my drinking would subside. I was no longer in direct practice with children, families, and vulnerable adults. There was no more secondary trauma. On top of that, I was teaching social workers to work with families dealing with addiction. How cognitively dissonant is that? By that time, I drank alone, one of the signs of a "high-functioning" drinker. I was going to great lengths to hide my drinking from my family, friends, and colleagues. It was so incredibly exhausting trying to keep up the facade.

Yesterday, I shared my one-year sober anniversary with my director. She told me how proud she was of me. We talked about creating a curriculum addressing potential alcohol abuse for social workers. It was liberating. How great is it I have a director I could share this with?

***

One of the recurring themes I see as I continue to do the work is how important "being of service to others" is on our sobriety journey. Traver Boehm (an amazing human—look him up) said you need to ask yourself, "Where does my talent intersect with what the world needs?" [36]

When we are of service to others, when we are kind and supportive, we produce endorphins, those wonderful "feel-good" chemicals in our brain. Helping others can lower anxiety and depression because it keeps you in the present. I know for me that being of service to others takes me out of my own head on those messy days when doubt and uncertainty happen. I see so many people in the recovery community supporting, encouraging, lifting each other up. That makes my heart happy. I know that every person I help strengthens my own recovery and keeps me moving forward.

***

Early this year, I did an exercise in the We Are the Luckiest course where I took a "shame inventory." There are two kinds of shame. Applied shame is given to you from the outside, from other people in your life, things that are not true, things that you internalize. My applied shame list included: "you're too loud," "you ask too many questions," "your personality is too big," "you need to act more like a lady," "an A isn't good enough," "you're almost pretty [wow]," "you're too emotional, too irrational," "you like everyone."

The other type of shame is authentic shame.

"Authentic shame helps you to live a value-driven life. It acts like a curb, nudging you back to alignment with your deepest sense of integrity." [37] —Karla McClaren

It happens when you have broken the code of your character. Like my drinking did. Both kinds of shame are important to understand in sobriety because feeling shame isn't always a bad thing. It can be a tool to effect positive change.

***

"There is a feeling of being cursed that comes from having an alcoholic mother, a curse that one can never shake off—it's as if someone forgot to give you the essential manual to life." [38]—Ann Dowsett Johnston

This is true for me. I knew growing up that something wasn't right, but I didn't realize my family's problem was alcohol. As a child, I had no words or understanding of what was going on or what my feelings really were. I just knew that things often felt "off," and I developed anxiety over wondering which mom was going to show up when I came home from school. It was pure craziness in my family because often, the best and the worst of times were one right after the other.

I remember daydreaming about being in a different family and immediately dismissed the thought because my brothers were everything to me. I know now that, for most of my adult life I have been seeking approval from others, almost losing myself in the process. I know that what hurts you at eight, hurts you at 68, unless you do something about it. What a complete gift sobriety and doing the work has been for me, my husband, my children, and my grandkids. I am finally one authentic me. One partner. One mother. Something my mother never had the opportunity to become.

***

I have been reading about how losing your parents early in life can affect your ability to form intimate relationships, and that there is a higher probability of turning to alcohol or substance abuse to cope. This explains the years of feeling like I missed out on so much.

Brains are still developing up to the age of 26, and it's difficult to grieve and grow at the same time. I had the double whammy of my mother's drinking and of the possibility of her making amends dying right along with her. So, besides the dysfunction growing up, I lost my limited but important cheerleading section. My parents were gone when I married, bought my first house, had three more children, put on my studio's first dance recital, earned my bachelor's and graduate degrees. My sounding board was missing. When so many of my friends were being parented well into their thirties, I felt lost and incomplete. "Am I doing this adult thing right? Would Bill and Margaret be proud of my accomplishments?"

I have been so uncomfortable going to my husband's family almost every holiday because that's when I missed my parents the most, when I felt the most alone. I was always super-anxious the day of these gatherings and often hit the wine as soon as I arrived. Sometimes even before I got there.

This first year of sobriety, I have leaned on my adult children, brothers, and good friends to fill those grandstand seats and it feels comfortable. I feel such belonging. I choose to be with my people for the holidays and my husband respects my choices. He would much rather have a sober wife.

***

I want to share something very special with you that I would never have attempted to do over my last years of drinking. It may seem like a little thing, but it was so big for me, so out of my comfort zone. I reached out to a friend I hadn't seen or heard from in decades. We were roommates in our twenties. Best friends. We met at an ice rink at the Sun Valley Mall in Concord, California, and instantly became inseparable. We did everything together. We partied, we skied, we played ice hockey, went to hockey games, played Santa and Mrs. Claus for the Oakland Seals Professional Hockey Team, got lost in the snow on Mount Hood in Oregon in a Volkswagen Beetle. We cried, we laughed, we took care of each other. We tortured our roommate. She was maid of honor at my wedding [Ed. note: My second of three.] Eventually, we lost touch.

I couldn't get Gretchen off my mind, so a few weeks ago, I reached out to her, and she responded. We talked for a couple hours on the phone and planned to meet for lunch the following Friday. It was as if no time had passed. We talked, we laughed, and we cried for three and a half hours. We cannot wait to see each other again. It was effortless and beautiful. Tears are flowing as I'm writing this. Being my most authentic self gave me the courage and the confidence to reach out to her—and what a gift it is to be reconnected. I am over the moon that I overcame my fear. The payoff is priceless.

***

Over this past year, my list of things-I-want-more-than-drinking grew—God, my marriage, my brothers, my friends (although some didn't make that list and that's okay because I have made many new ones in this community), my writing, teaching, my integrity, self-esteem, self-worth, and purpose. On July 11, 2019, I would have told you none of these things were remotely possible. I was dying. Yes, I was on that trajectory. Yet, here I am.

***

Yesterday morning, I woke up feeling extremely anxious and overwhelmed, and was leaking tears for no apparent reason. I know right now I have a bit of an over-committed teaching schedule this month, and I'm not the biggest fan of virtual teaching. As you might guess, I thrive on the energy in the classroom. I did some box breathing, recited my Surrender Novena prayer, and read through my latest journal where I came across this AA affirmation:

"Your worst day sober is better than your best day drinking." [39]

Immediately, I felt better. I'm learning to sit with my feelings, and I'm comforted with the thought that I always have the option of reaching out to a sober friend through a call, a text, or a post. No matter how I feel today, or even at a particular moment, I know that tomorrow will be different. I know bad days are temporary.

***

We don't really learn much when things are going well. The lessons we learn come from pain and being right outside our comfort zone.

"As much as it might hurt and as much as we might want to turn back the hands of time, we should never regret the decisions we made no matter what or where they lead us in life." [40] —Laura McKowen

We grow spiritually, mentally, and emotionally when we experience pain and/or setbacks. I sometimes look at others' success and compare my life with theirs. But then I think of my son Matthew, a person of very few words, who said to me: "Mom, if you hadn't lost your first child, our sister, none of us would have happened—me, Lindsay and Brett wouldn't be here right now." That put it all into perspective for me. Thank you, my wise son. For sure, I wouldn't be here, posting every day. There is a reason for everything. Nothing is wasted. In doing this work, I no longer regret the years it took me to get here.

"Being fully human is not about feeling happy, it's about feeling everything. I learned that I will never be free from pain, but I could be free from the fear of pain and that was enough." [41] —Glennon Doyle

***

I was asked the other day what my plans are for continuing my sober journey in year two. Simple. I am committed to protecting my sobriety at all costs. Fiercely. I will continue to navigate being alcohol free in a world that, for the most part, is not. I have armed myself with all kinds of habits that would make it extremely difficult to go back to that old life—posting every day, writing, surrendering, having morning/nightly rituals, exercising, carefully recruiting sober allies, committing to being a lifelong learner.

> "If you're proud [of being alcohol free], you'll develop all sorts of habits to maintain it. Once your pride gets involved, you'll fight tooth and nail to maintain it. Then, when your behavior and identity are fully aligned, you are no longer pursuing behavior change. You are simply acting like the person you already believe yourself to be."
> —James Clear [42]

***

I know that the further the distance I am from my last drink, the easier it could be to romance the wine glass. Doing so would be to travel down a very dangerous road. Without the daily work I put into sobriety, I run the risk of forgetting just how bad my drinking was – the inability to stop after one, drinking alone, lying, blackouts, disturbed sleep, chronic fatigue, depression, anxiety, hangovers, and outbursts of anger. I know there is no safe level of alcohol for me. Research suggests there is no safe level of alcohol consumption for anyone.

There may be some people who are successful in moderation. For me, the empirical evidence of my drinking history is quite clear - moderation would turn into relapse. I stopped looking for what Laura McKowen calls "the third door", one that gives us a life with the upside of drinking without any of the downsides. This third door does not exist for me. I tried that many times and failed. I can never forget. I will never forget. A permanent commitment to abstinence means I no longer have to fight a battle with moderation; but rather devote myself entirely to sobriety.

***

I am sitting here, with my steaming cup of Kauai Island Sunrise coffee, reflecting on my years of suffering with my secret-yet-not-so-secret drinking life. I'm still blown away that, professionally, I managed to pull it off like I did for so long. Simply amazing. Maybe simply lucky. I think about how those secrets kept me so very sick for the last several years. And through a lot of denial, anger, and tears, I finally had the "aha" moment that I couldn't DIY my way through sobriety by just reading a hundred books and listening to podcasts. I had to do so much more, and it has been no joke. Certainly, it has been the most difficult thing I have done besides childbirth and burying my daughter. This is probably my favorite Laura McKowen quote:

"Sobriety forced a closeness to myself and to life that was at first, excruciating. It burned and it burned and it burned. But in the ashes from burning all the things I was not, I found her. I found me. And then I could finally be found by others. It was my opening. It led me straight to everything I always wanted but never knew how to get. And it had to break me. There was no other way. There is no other way for any of us." [43]

There was certainly no other way for me.

***

For about ten years before I stopped drinking, I increasingly suffered from insomnia and sleep apnea issues that I blamed on aging and the secondary trauma of being a child welfare social worker. I never thought that my drinking had anything to do with not being able to sleep. In fact, I drank wine to help me sleep. I spent thousands of dollars on sleep. My doctor prescribed Xanax and Ambien. And, of course, despite warnings against it, I was taking these prescription drugs right along with my wine. Taking Ambien could have its own separate post. Getting off Ambien, which I successfully did about five years ago, was a nightmare; it was much more difficult than quitting alcohol. I don't think I slept for an entire week. And when I didn't have the Ambien, my drinking increased. Pure insanity.

I suffered through sleep studies where they attached a gazillion wires all over my head and body and then expected me to sleep in a bed that wasn't mine. Not to mention that women of my age are prone to making several trips to the restroom at night. That required the detaching and reattaching of all those wires. And I could hear the "sleep monitors" talking and laughing in the other room through my earphones.

I recently spent over $6,000 on Invisaligns to widen my jaw to open my airway.

Here, of course, is the kicker: Without alcohol, I can sleep! Imagine that. I tuck myself into bed sober, listen to my 22-minute Insight Timer Yoga Nidra by Jennifer Piercy, and I rarely hear the end before I drift off. Being able to sleep is incentive enough to stay sober.

***

More on blackouts: Having blackouts was probably the worst kind of shame I experienced when I was drinking. The aftermath from blackouts left me with self-loathing and anxiety that would last for days. Not being able to remember what I said or what I did the night before was its own special kind of hell. Blackouts were so confusing and frightening for my husband because, when I was in one, he could tell something was wrong, but most of the time, I was still functioning somewhat normally. I don't know how many times he made excuses for me by telling people I was just "tired." I could walk, hold conversations, have sex, get into arguments and, the most frightening thing, get in a car and drive. I would either remember nothing or maybe bits and pieces if I was having a gray-out. (In gray-outs, you can remember some of what happened, but not all.) I read Sarah Hepola's book *Blackout*, and just recently listened to Annie Grace's podcast #304 on the subject. (I highly recommend both.) Hepola writes that you are likely to experience blackouts when you drink too fast and drink on an empty stomach. This totally explains why I experienced more blackouts at the end of my drinking career. By that time, I was often slamming my wine because I was hiding or sneaking it, and I was notorious for not eating when I drank. Blackouts increase if you take Xanax with alcohol. Check. Women are much more susceptible to blackouts than men because we metabolize alcohol at a slower rate.

***

Recently, we had our four-year-old twin grandkids up to the cabin for the weekend. They were playing with a couple of their favorite toys, the ice cream truck and the hot dog stand. (Check out Our Generation toys from Target. We have a camper, ice cream truck, veterinary clinic, Christmas sleigh, picnic table, fruit/vegetable stand, and a movie theater, too.) All the grandkids spend hours playing with these toys. I was listening to them and they were pretending to serve beer with the hot dogs. At four years of age. And even though their parents model appropriate and moderate use of alcohol. (Is there really such a thing?) It makes you think how normalized drinking is in our society. It's crazy how being sober makes you notice everything.

***

Yesterday, I heard a keynote speaker, Maria Escobar, at our National Coaching Conference give a presentation on brain functioning, particularly about how our amygdala and our prefrontal cortex (PFC) communicate to recognize threats and process emotions. Our amygdala is the primitive, reptilian part of our brain that constantly scans for threats. It doesn't think; it only learns. The PFC manages complex information and sees possibilities; it's creative, it reasons, it figures things out. It's the thinking part of the brain.

I was curious about what is the effect of alcohol on these two brain parts. The amygdala, an almond-shaped collection of nuclei found deep within the temporal lobe, can be viewed as a sort of driver behind emotion. When we drink too much, the emotional cues that signal threats aren't being processed in the brain normally because the "drunk" amygdala isn't responding as it should. Alcohol inhibits the interaction of the amygdala with the PFC and impairs how we respond to emotions and threats. Sound familiar? We have emotions for a reason.

Drinking works to temporarily quiet those emotions and prolongs the struggle because they don't get processed and worked through. The more we drink, the more anxious we become, and the cycle perpetuates. And, if we aren't connected to ourselves, we certainly cannot be connected to others. Without drinking, I can be a present, functioning human being, ready to take on life's many ups and downs. I can pay attention to my emotions and tell my amygdala, "Hey, I got this. I feel you. I can take it from here."

***

Yesterday, at the same conference, I attended a workshop called "Conversational Cocktails" (haha, how appropriate) with Roe Couture DeSaro. I believe we can create or destroy connections with people with the words we use. Words can drive our behavior. Words change worlds. When someone tells us what we need or have to do (like getting sober), it can create resistance, inaction, and/or mistrust.

I know that when my husband told me I needed or had to do something about my drinking (or else), it only pushed my behavior further underground, and my drinking went rogue. I think if he had approached me differently, expressed how worried he was, I might have listened to him. Maybe if he had asked me, "What do you think could happen in your life, our lives, if you stop drinking?" Many scenarios and possibilities could emerge. The list could be endless, right? He would come from a place of not knowing the answer, a place of curiosity, of non-judgment, which creates high trust. (BTW, we are working on doing more of this type of communicating now.) Our conversations have switched from an "I" centered position to "We".

This is the magic of our recovery community. We start to feel that curious, inquisitive nature in each other and we listen to connect. We learn compassion, which is to hold space for each other without judgment. We open our hearts and minds for mutual success.

***

It has been crazy wonderful how every presentation and workshop I attended at my coaching conference this week had me think about how relatable the topics were to my sober journey and even more so because this week's topic for the Sober Sis Alcohol-Free Living course I am taking is "connection." There are no coincidences, right? (And did I mention that this was my first experience as a presenter in a national conference, speaking on the hijacking of the amygdala?) In this second year of sobriety, I'm finding myself sitting back more and talking less. (My husband may call "bullshit" on that.) When I was drinking, words would pour out of me, and I didn't know how others were receiving them. My mind was often too altered to care. Now, sans drinking, I listen to connect or understand, rather than to respond. I love being the observer. And I know people can feel it in their bodies if you are truly listening to connect.

> "When we do that, we connect through our heart and our pre-frontal cortex. Our centers of empathy, compassion, openness, and receptivity to other's point of view are activated." [44]—Judith Glaser/*Conversational Intelligence.*

I can also listen for what is not being said as well. In conversations like this, both people receive a colossal hit of the feel-good chemical oxytocin. Everything happens through conversation.

***

At a little over 13 months sober, I'm just beginning to let my guard down with my husband. I don't think he is aware of just how disconnected I can feel from him because, from his perspective, he "has his wife back." And for sure, we rarely argue anymore; there is trust and peace and laughter in our home again. Paul doesn't look at sobriety in the same way I do. He shouldn't have to. Alcohol was never his thing. But I don't feel like I am "back"; I feel like I have been reborn. I have put in so much work to get here that I sometimes I feel I have left him back at the station. Does that make any sense? And I really do fully appreciate the unfairness to him.

Today, I am re-committing to working harder on our communication and our relationship. One of the keynote speakers at the conference last week talked about Judith Glaser's term "double-clicking"—certainly a concept my financial analyst husband can relate to.

> "Double-clicking with the intention to share and discover what the other person feels and means can be transformative for how you approach conversations. It opens up a safer space for you and the other person to connect more deeply and purposefully." [45]

I know that unless Paul and I learn to double-click and dig deeper to understand each other, we will continue to assume we are communicating and that's not enough for me, not enough for us, anymore.

***

In the first few months of my sobriety, I had some strong ideas on how my husband needed to support me, and when he didn't meet those expectations, I sincerely thought our marriage was beyond fixing. Although my drinking had exacerbated the problems in our marriage and most definitely contributed to some unhealthy patterns of communication, they existed long before I used alcohol to cope. I mean, geez, we've been married for 34 years. Many times, I drank because of the way I let his words make me feel. Conflicts stayed unresolved and festered. The more upset he got, the more I drank. I know that my sobriety changed everything in our relationship because, although my alcohol-free lifestyle has been a tremendous source of pride for him, it has also been confusing because I have finally been able to set clear boundaries for how I want and need to be treated as an equal partner. I see him looking at me and wondering, "Who is this woman I am married to, who no longer views people pleasing as a priority, who expresses her needs in a healthy way and basically doesn't take shit from anyone—including me—anymore?" I know it has taken a lot of years to get to where we are now, and we both need to give our relationship time and grace to heal so that we can move in a forward direction. I am so grateful to be sober and to do just that.

***

Looking back over this first year, I realize how much I have leaned on women and men in our community who have hung in there with their significant others despite the many barriers and challenges. I really wanted my marriage to work.

"I think it's incredibly important to look for people who have stayed in their relationships if that's your goal. It's very easy for people who aren't in a partnership or have left theirs to tell you, 'Just leave, they will never understand.'" [46] —Megan Peters

One of my dear friends, Karen, advised me to not make any major decisions in my first year of sobriety, and this advice has served me well. It took so much pressure off me, and I have been able to concentrate on healing and getting well.

***

I seem to be on a relationship posting roll. So, let's continue. Since the start of our 35-year relationship, I have allowed my husband's words to have the power to cut me like a knife. During the last few years of my drinking career, I let those words justify my drinking entire bottles of wine in a single setting. I have also witnessed my husband be in so much emotional pain over my drinking, it has reduced him to tears. It often felt hopeless for both of us. Social pain releases some of the same chemicals as physical pain. I broke his heart many times.

In doing this work, the way I take in his words is so different now and I try to listen to connect, rather than listen for rejection. Paul's words can still hurt, but I now have the tools to take a pause before I react to them, because often the interpretation I give to them isn't reality.

Judith Glaser's list of five barriers to connection has been so helpful in my journey:

- The first involves an assumption that others see what we see, feel what we feel, and think what we think.
- The second is the failure to realize that fear, trust, and distrust change how we see and interpret reality and how we talk about it.
- The third is the inability to stand in each other's shoes when we are fearful or upset.
- The fourth is the assumption that we remember what others say, when we actually remember what we think others say.
- The fifth is the assumption that meaning resides in the speaker, when in fact, it resides in the listener. Words do change worlds. [47]

**

How in the world did I ever wake up to find myself in a place where alcohol became more important than my relationships and health? I'm sure many of you have asked yourselves that same question. It's simple, really. Our brains are always seeking homeostasis, the path of least resistance. We default to the familiar. And, for years, coming home and drinking wine was my familiar. The only way we can change our behavior is to get uncomfortable. I was listening to Laura McKowen last week, and she talked about Dr. Andrew Huberman's work in this area. He says we only grow when we create agitation and push through it. Agitation barely describes how I felt in those early days of sobriety. That's where change happens—right outside your comfort zone—and everything seems new for a very good reason. (It is.) And make no mistake—when we are trying to accomplish something difficult, and getting sober is really fucking difficult, we lay down thicker neural networks. This means, with practice, our skill of not drinking becomes more potent than our skill of drinking.

✳✳✳

Recently, I had a vivid flashback of my brother Jerry and my sister-in-law-who-is-more-like-a-sister, Linda, walking into the kitchen at our cabin where they witnessed me chugging wine straight from the wine bottle. They said nothing at that moment, but Linda had tears in her eyes. Her only sister, her only sibling, died from cirrhosis years ago. I was full of anxiety the entire night. Linda and Jerry had a serious talk with me in the morning. More tears. They were worried. I begged them not to tell Paul, and they didn't.

That afternoon, things went from bad to worse. Paul asked everyone what they wanted to drink, and Jerry said, "I'll have a vodka tonic." I went into total panic. You see, I drank what was left in the bottle the night before, replaced it with water and hadn't had the opportunity to buy another. I had to pull my brother aside and tell him one more low life thing I had done.

That was a year before my last drink. Until now, I'd forgotten about the vodka part altogether. The wine incident was bad enough. So, although this memory was a painful one, I am taking away two things: I'm no longer that person (my brother, as he says it, has his sister back); and my brain is clearly recovering from alcohol because I can remember more. Another neuroscience lesson: When you stop drinking, there is an increase in the volume of the hippocampus, a brain region involved in many memory functions and which is associated with memory improvement.

✳✳✳

I know that out of every tool I have learned to get and stay AF, surrendering has been my greatest sober superpower. On July 12, 2019, I literally found myself on my knees, on the verge of losing almost everything I loved. In my most profound pain, I heard and felt that voice saying, "You are done—and you will be okay." In that moment, I felt a deep sense of calm. I was consumed in pain, yet I recognized the truth in what I heard. I told my daughter this, and she was understandably extremely doubtful. She had heard it all

118

before. But I knew in that moment, I had drunk my last glass of wine.

Surrendering has become the cornerstone of my sobriety.

"Surrendering puts us in a position to be at peace [with] what is. It puts the past behind us, and it opens up our hearts, minds and spirits to the present. By surrendering our old messy imperfectness, we allow a new version of ourselves to emerge. It is the death of what isn't working and has not worked in a long time. It is the birth of something new and fresh and gives us a chance to fulfill the potential we know we have deep down inside of us."[48] —Carly Benson

I start every day with my Surrender Novena prayers. They have become a part of my non-negotiable morning ritual. Thank you, Susan Keeley. She gave them to me a couple years ago; I said them for a while, and then I put them in the drawer. Now I carry them everywhere with me, and one of my biggest joys is when I can send them to others.

Without surrendering, nothing else makes sense in my life. It is the difference between giving up and giving it over to God. Surrendering keeps me in that humble and teachable place and makes all things possible. It makes living my life possible.

***

A bit more on surrendering. Surrendering has allowed me to be vulnerable, to have the courage to seek opportunities that are leading me closer to my authentic self. I think back to last year and years prior, after so many attempts to quit drinking on my own. I convinced myself that I was in control, that I had all the answers. It was easy, right? All I had to do was stop drinking. After all, I managed several periods of sobriety in the past. I never lost a day's work because of my drinking. (Well, except for that one time at that conference in San Diego I was being paid to attend when I spent one morning in the hotel room throwing up.) Never mind those gray-outs and blackouts that increasingly filled me with anxiety. As Dr. Phil would ask, "How's that working for you?" When we surrender, we allow for strength to come from sources other than ourselves. We give up our need to be right. We give up our need to control everything. And now, my vulnerability has become my ticket to freedom. I am no longer living small.

> "You're off to great places. Today is your day. Your mountain is waiting. Now get on your way." [49] —Dr. Seuss

***

One of my sober sisters, Nathalie, talked about how she and her French-Canadian sisters could write a book about their alcohol-induced shenanigans of the past. I recently had lunch with a best friend I reconnected with, and we spent three hours laughing and crying hysterically about the same thing. I will spare my husband and adult children and you the details. There are plenty of memories I would like to erase, but some of them were hilarious. I wouldn't have been able to deal with the severity of some of the things I've done without humor. Humor is one of my core values. It has given me the ability to write about shameful, painful, I-hate-my-fucking-guts things that I thought I could never tell to another soul.

When I can share my experiences, there is almost always another person who says, "I did that, too." That connection, that feeling of belonging, makes things better and hope grows.

> "First of all, let's be real, a lot of things we did while drinking were just plain funny, but beyond that, the laughter is a release valve, allowing us to recognize the ridiculousness of ourselves, the thinking alongside the very painful memories. And the connection it creates, laughing with others about things that perhaps the rest of the world wouldn't find very amusing." [50]—Janelle Hanchett

***

I have written about this before, but I wanted to share how the art of saying "no" has played, and continues to play, a major role in my sobriety. Laura McKowen writes:

> "It's about being comfortable with your no and not going into a song and dance apology." [51]

I love this. I still want to explain my no's. Not being able to say "no" was a huge drinking trigger for me, because I would be so annoyed at myself for not saying it when I should have or needed to. I cannot tell you how saying "no" kept me from drinking so many times this past year. "No, I am not going to that concert. I just don't like all those crowds and noise and standing for hours." "No, I am going to skip the Super Bowl Party." "No, I think I'll pass on that wine-tasting trip." "No, I have attended a lifetime of baby or wedding showers. Where can I send my gift?"

I can say "no" with an alternative solution, like I did a couple days ago with my daughter-in-law. "No, I can't help you move, but I would be glad to pay for a housekeeper and please give me a list of some things you need for the new house." She was thrilled, and we both got our needs met. Saying "no" is self-care and helps to keep me alcohol free and at peace. And saying "no" doesn't always mean "never"; sometimes saying "no" simply means "not now." You can still be a good person with a kind heart and say "no" sometimes.

***

When I was nine years old, I was riding in the back seat of my parents' car on a road trip through Wyoming and Montana. We had just left Yellowstone Park. My dad was a national park fanatic. We would drive hours and days to visit them. During this trip, my older brothers were out on their own and my younger brother hadn't been born yet. My mom turned to me and said, "I need to take a nap. Watch your dad's head and make sure he doesn't fall asleep." Mind you, my dad is driving the fucking car we are riding in! Whhhhaaaatttt? And, of course, a few miles in, I see my dad's head start to fall towards his left shoulder accompanied by a snoring sound, and I yell at him: "Dad, wake up! You're falling asleep!" He wasn't happy and denied that he was drifting off. As a child welfare social worker, I thank God that CPS was non-existent at that time.

This has become one of those "remember when …?" stories, bringing much laughter at family gatherings. It was also where I learned that saying "no" was selfish, and the thought never occurred to me that this was an inappropriate responsibility to put on a nine-year-old child. Nor was it appropriate for my mom to pull me into arguments or incidents between her and my dad. No, Mom, I really didn't want to know about that time Dad almost choked you. Or about the time the lipstick on my dad's forehead wasn't yours. I experienced and was exposed to adult issues for which I had no words or understanding. And I was too young to understand that most of it was fueled by alcohol. With the help of my psychologist, I am learning to forgive my mother for using me as her marital therapist. I am re-parenting myself in a way that I missed as a child, and part of that is realizing that saying "no" isn't selfish at all; it's self-preservation.

***

I was having lunch with my brother Bob the other day and he reminded me of an incident I had completely forgotten about. He was about five and I was 15. We were in Dad's "boat" of an Oldsmobile Delta 88 driving down the highway on a hot summer day to go waterskiing at Lake Berryessa. He threw his cigarette out the window, and it blew back through the rear seat window and landed in Bob's lap and it was still lit! I screamed for my dad to stop the car, that Bob was on fire. Dad pulled over, got out, opened my brother's passenger door, and put the cigarette out with his beer. He got back into the driver's seat and drove on like nothing ever happened.

That boat of an automobile became my first car—a bribe from my parents to make me feel better about the divorce and traumatic move to be closer to my mother's sister. I remember that big burn hole in the back seat. Crazy-ass family.

I walk almost every morning. I woke up on Tuesday and it was raining and cold, and I did something I rarely do: I decided I wouldn't walk because, I told myself, I needed extra time to prepare for a class I was teaching that day. (I curse you, COVID, and this continued online instruction.) Walking is a non-negotiable activity in my AF journey. If I miss one day, I get back into it as quickly as possible.

> "Missing one [day of walking, journaling/writing, saying my Surrender Novenas] happens, but I'm not going to miss two in a row … I can't be perfect, but I can avoid a second lapse. The first mistake is never the one that ruins you. It is the spiral of repeated mistakes that follows. Missing once is an accident. Missing twice is the start of a new habit." [52]—James Clear

I work hard to avoid getting a case of the "fuck-its." Even on days I don't get in my full walk, I try to do a smaller one. My sobriety depends on it.

***

I get a lot of messages from people who ask how I have stayed alcohol free. After so many day ones I can't possibly count (crash diets just don't work, right?), the difference this time is the pure grit I have put into living a sober life. I have very few cracks in my routine. My commitment to wake up every day and not drink has completely changed the way I think about myself.

You can stop drinking with sheer willpower alone, but your willpower is limited, and when it runs out, you risk going back to drinking.

> "Gritty people don't skip workouts, or fail to meet a daily goal, nor do they shirk responsibilities. They show up for themselves every single day, even when it sucks." [53] —James Clear

Walking has been one of those habits that has literally changed my brain chemistry. I didn't do so well last year during winter. This year, I have lots of miles under my belt, and I have ordered warm walking gear. I plan to kick winter's butt.

I keep this Post It on my bathroom mirror to remind me of how important my new sober habits are: "No matter how many mistakes you make or how slow your progress, you are still way ahead of everyone else who isn't trying."

***

Yesterday, a student in my virtual social work class was having an awful morning. COVID has made it next to impossible for social workers to do their job, which is to protect our most vulnerable population—children and elders. Many of them are juggling work and family. Virtual education has started. Even though I couldn't feel the energy in the room like I can in the classroom, I could see the tension and sadness on a particular student's face. So, I stopped teaching and we all just listened to her story. She was trying to juggle new motherhood with work at home, and she was in tears. All the students in the class rallied around their co-worker, lifting her up, holding space by wrapping her with encouragement, compassion, and love. And, at that moment, I was overwhelmed with gratitude for the gift of being totally present for her and for the entire class.

Before I got sober, I might have come to class with a hangover, maybe missing the opportunity entirely.

Two years ago, I received an outstanding service award out of 1,750 colleagues. The award felt fraudulent and undeserving. I was tortured on the inside, wondering when my directors, colleagues, and students would see through me and my complete hypocrisy of teaching social workers how to work with children and families whose lives have been affected by addiction. You would think I would stop drinking. Or cut way down (too late for that). Nope. That would take close to another year.

Drinking had become such a nightly ritual after teaching all day. The first thing I would usually do would be to stop at the store on the way home from class and pick up a bottle of sauvignon blanc. Twist tops, of course. I deserved it, right?

On other days, I knew what teaching tasks needed to be done before I poured a giant glass of wine, which ones could be put off (I don't teach every day), and which ones I could accomplish while drinking.

When I traveled to teach, there were the hotels that offered wine happy hours and I would take the elevator down to the lobby right at six to get my free glasses of shitty chardonnay, sometimes in addition to the bottle I bought. I planned my drinking around teaching, often leaving my family out of the equation. I blamed being tired on teaching. Paul told me that if teaching was too much for me, I should quit. It wasn't the teaching.

My students are getting an instructor who is fully present, clear-headed, available. They deserve nothing less. I am grateful that I had eight months of sobriety when COVID hit. Working from home might have been way more of a challenge than it already is.

I thank God for my sober life. Again, and again and again.

***

The Enneagram has become another path to self-discovery on my sober journey.

The Enneagram is born out of Jungian psychology and the exploration of archetypes and the shadow self. Similar to a Myers-Briggs personality test, the Enneagram is a tool used for understanding self and others, but it investigates deeper beneath the personality to explore the unconscious human binaries of fear and desire, and stressors and strengths, to optimize healthier levels of self-awareness and improve understanding of others. By understanding more about the complexity of our everyday blind-spots, we can connect on deeper levels with ourselves and others to bring forward our true, authentic self instead of our protective fear-driven self. There are nine Enneagram types based on archetypes (and depending on sources referred to by different names, but you get the gist): Type 1: The Perfectionist; Type 2: The Helper; Type 3: The Achiever; Type 4: The Romantic; Type 5: The Observer; Type 6:

The Questioner; Type 7: The Entertainer; Type 8: The Challenger; Type 9: The Peacemaker.

I am a Type 7. Sevens are jacks-of-all-trades. They believe in possibility and are an endearing blend of charm and curiosity, suffused with a feeling of "hooray for tomorrow". Sevens are truth tellers (when they are sober) whose wisdom can be quick and inspiring. Sevens are joy bringers, and when they've truly discovered happiness, their enthusiasm and drive to share it with everyone by teaching others how to find it for themselves knows no limits (hence this book).

The downside is that Sevens can be prone to alcohol abuse—any addiction, really—because we don't like negativity and tend to run from pain, avoiding it at all costs. The last thing a Seven wants to feel is stuck. My Enneagram work has helped me to understand that my drinking was my way of numbing, to avoid darkness and painful emotions. With alcohol (and Xanax and Ambien), I could sidestep any wave of grief or sadness. "Excuse me, I don't do sadness. I do fun. I do funny. I make you laugh. I say outlandish, random things you would never dare to say out loud."

I still do all these things, only sober. My alcohol-free life has allowed me to sit with the myriad of emotions that flow through me daily, letting them come and go as they wish. Like cats.

***

This is totally random. (Of course, it is! I am a Seven.) One of the tools I use to unwind and/or destress is to cut up or slice fruits and veggies and put them into storage containers. The steady chop, chop, chop of my knife against the cutting board quiets my mind and soothes my soul. For real. My friends know this about me and often check in with me when they see or hear me chopping. "You're chopping. Are you okay?"

This activity is a perfect "wine-o'clock" alternative and helped me get through some intense cravings and feelings. Chopping encourages us to practice mindfulness by forcing our minds to concentrate on the task at hand, rather than on past or future problems. Then there is the bonus of having healthy food choices available. I am much more inclined to grab a cup of watermelon or berries or cucumbers instead of some carb-loaded, processed snack. I have become famous for my chili lime salsa. It's a total win-win situation.

My chopping has made it into The Luckiest Club's "Top 100 Things To Do Instead of Drinking" list. Ha!

***

I have been teaching about "Being versus Doing" in my coaching class for over six years, yet I didn't know how to just "be" in my own life. BEING takes us back to our simple existence. It is focused on the present moment and allows for reflection and thought of things that happen, rather than trying to affect the flow of things or events. DOING involves taking action and requires us to interact with our environment and other people to achieve a certain goal. Doing is easier than being because it gives us a sense (albeit often a false one) that we are in control of our lives and can feel like the more comfortable option.

> "Sometimes it's better to do nothing and to stay with our fears until a solution shows itself." [54] —Henneke

Certainly, there was no room for being in my life when I was drinking. I prided myself on being an excellent doer, but I was incapable of being when numbed out on alcohol. I have discovered there is such value in the balance of both. It is important to know when to be on the stage performing, and when to be on the balcony observing. Both are necessary for a balanced life.

> "You must give up the life you planned in order to have the life that is waiting for you." [55] —Joseph Campbell

***

On my morning walk yesterday, I came across a discarded mini bottle of New Amsterdam vodka on the ground. I couldn't believe that one little bottle could bring up so many feelings/emotions/

memories for me—shame, sadness, Maui ABC Stores where I used to buy them on vacay (because I couldn't have a good time in one of the most beautiful places on earth without booze, right?). I had compassion and empathy for the person who threw it there. No judgment. I ended my rollercoaster of feelings with relief and peace, knowing I am no longer part of the Secret Life of Mini Bottles.

[Mini bottles date back to 1862. States viewed them as either moving towards or away from moderation. They hit their golden age in the 1960s and 1970s and have made quite a comeback in current days. Mini bottles fit nicely into a woman's purse. They are easier to hide in trash bins. As a child, I remember seeing thousands of them displayed in a popular liquor store in Lake Tahoe and I was in total awe, not knowing they had the potential to destroy lives.]

***

Guess what? I LOVE going to bed now, because I am choosing to go to bed rather than waking up in the morning with little or no recollection of how I got there. I seriously drive my husband crazy because I cannot wait until it's time to go to bed. I usually get ready for bed about 9:00 (or earlier) with my nightly routine that often includes taking a peppermint eucalyptus Epsom salts bath before climbing into my bed and slipping between sheets sprayed with sea salt or lavender spray. Waking up sober has got to be the best feeling on the planet. It. Never. Gets. Old. Absent is waking up to those feelings of skyrocketing anxiety, guilt, or fog. No more what-the-fuck-did-I-do-last-night? mornings. There is only joy, freedom, gratitude. Delicious moments of silence (unless the dog of unusual size upstairs is pacing and anxiously barking to get his owners to take him out). There is extra time and energy to write, read, and reflect. And last, but certainly not least, there is peace.

***

Being divorced twice has been a source of great shame, guilt, and failure for me. I used to just cringe when anyone brought up the fact that I have been married three times. I had a boss who loved to bring this up in front of my co-workers. I have an ex-brother-in-law who promised to "expose" me if I didn't tell his mother I had been married before and had a child. What an asshole. I am a child of divorce. I broke my promise to myself that I would never get divorced. I never wanted that for my own children whose lives it has affected not only by divorce, but by growing up in a blended family with all the challenges that go with it.

But yesterday, my heart was full. My son Brett brought his dad, stepmom, and uncle to spend Labor Day weekend at our cabin where they will hang out, play golf, and kayak. Brett called last night, so full of pride that he could do this for his dad. And I love how comfortable my ex and his partner are with going up there. It says a lot about them. It feels good. It feels right. This would have never happened with my parents because my mom never got over my dad leaving her. She gave bitter a whole additional dimension. Doing this work has helped me to drop the shame and guilt and be grateful because my ex and I have been able to successfully co-parent our three amazing kids. My kids are so lucky to have Michelle as a stepmother. I couldn't pick a better person to be another mother to my children.

***

Yesterday, I had lunch with one of my best friends, Gretchen, at an amazing restaurant, Bella Sienna, in Benicia that looks out over the San Francisco Bay. As you may recall, Gretchen and I reconnected after being apart for almost four decades. She was maid of honor at one of my weddings. A few years later, life happened. We lost touch.

Reconnecting with Gretchen will continue to be one of the greatest gifts of being AF. Without sobriety, I wouldn't have reached out to her. I thought about her so many times. For the last several years, I was so unhappy with myself that I didn't think I had anything to offer our friendship. I accomplished a lot in those 30-plus years we had been apart, but I didn't think I was worthy of rekindling this relationship. I found myself isolating or feeling like I was letting down the friends I currently had. I was in a place where I'd done so many inappropriate things, told so many lies, I believed I was irredeemable. I didn't know who I was. But I know now.

I have discovered that some friendships have an emotional longevity that is resilient to dormant periods, even very long ones. We both took the chance that our reconnection might have produced an afternoon of memories only to part again, feeling better for having connected. And that would have been okay. It ended up being so much more than that. We both marvel that the old chemistry is there, deepened by our experience in between.

I love you, G. I am beyond grateful we found each other again.

"A good friend is a connection to life—a tie to the past, a road to the future, the key to sanity in a totally insane world." [56] —Lois Wyse

***

I am sure that with COVID, widespread wildfires, and a particularly emotionally charged election, the year 2020 will qualify as "totally insane." It will become synonymous with "mind-blowingly fucked up" for all the reasons I've mentioned thus far, but it has also been a silver lining in my life.

***

I am sitting here, early morning, enjoying everything about my coffee, reflecting on my second AF Labor Day, while four of my grandkids, two sets of twins, ages four and eight, are asleep, huddled together as twins tend to do. My husband made a comment last night about how much he enjoys having the kids over now that I'm not drinking. He said I am so much more focused and relaxed. Agreed. I feel like I have single-handedly discovered the Three Ps of Grandparent Sleepovers—PATIENCE: I practically have an endless amount because I'm not hungover or sleep deprived. PREPARATION: I have all food prepared, meals planned, snacks available, drinking cups "sharpi'd" with their names, activities, toys and rainbow bath bombs. PRESENT: I know the grandkids can sense things have been different in our home because the tension is gone. It's peaceful. Predictable. As soon as they see me, they run up and administer ginormous hugs. They know they can trust me to be the same person. Every. Single. Time. Sober grandmothers ROCK!

Oh, and the littlies were pretend playing with the new vet clinic toy, and I overheard them asking each other repeatedly, "Do you have the hand sanitizer?" Another "COVIDism" that was kind of funny and sad at the same time.

***

I discovered something completely cool to do with my grandkids: conversation cards. They help me and other grownups (did I really refer to myself as a grownup?) share thoughtful discussions about emotions, feelings, growth, imagination, mindfulness, kindness, resilience, core values, and gratitude with your little and not-so-little family members. There are questions like, "What made your brain grow today?" "What is your favorite way to feel calm?" "What is one quality you look for in a friend?" "What is something that makes you really mad?" "Pretend the internet doesn't exist. How would you communicate with people from different parts of the world?" "What would you do if you saw your friend stealing something in the store?"

What does this have to do with being sober? In the US, we teach our five- and six-year-olds hundreds of sight words, but none of them describe emotions or feelings. We rarely teach them to name their feelings, talk about them, or deal with them. Maybe if we do more of that, they won't grow up thinking they need to numb out those feelings with alcohol or drugs. Cards like these are one way to equip our kids with tools for dealing with their emotions in healthy, productive ways. Our grandkids, even the four-year-olds, love these cards and beg to play. Their answers can be quite hilarious. And it's a great way to pull in the teenagers, who can be challenging to engage. (The preceding sentence was the ultimate understatement.) There is nothing like sitting around the fire, roasting marshmallows for s'mores and having these conversations. Unless it's going to bed at 9:00.

***

I lied so much when I was drinking, it became second nature to me. Paul would ask me how much I'd had to drink. I would often deny I'd had anything, or I might say, "I just had two glasses." (A lie.) Did you drink some of my bourbon? "Of course not. I hate bourbon. You know I would never touch that stuff" (A half-lie. I DO hate bourbon, but if it was the only thing standing, I wouldn't hesitate.) "Oh, the kids must have drunk that when they were up last time." (That happened once, or maybe twice—big pathetic lie.) The lying became a twisted game where I found satisfaction in just getting away with it. Fourteen months into my sobriety, I still find telling the truth to be difficult at times (mostly about the most insignificant things) because lying had become such a habit.

Yesterday, I stopped myself from texting my hair stylist asking to reschedule my appointment because we were going to be out of town (truth). The whole truth was that last month she didn't feel comfortable doing my hair because of COVID, so I went to another stylist, and I didn't need her to do my hair now. I felt guilty and didn't want her to be upset. Ridiculous. I have been going to her for years and she would totally understand. Which, of course, she did when I texted her the whole truth/nothing but the truth. (You know the drill.) This may seem like a small, insignificant thing, but to me it's the residual of my dishonest days of drinking. Bending the truth to spare someone's feelings is still lying. I now practice intentional honesty daily, pausing to ask myself, "Is what I am about to say the truth?" A friend calls it personal integrity. Or alignment. Sometimes it's more than not lying, but a deeper understanding and living the truest truth. And sometimes we don't even know ourselves, and it takes some time to figure it out. I call it a path to freedom.

***

Added to the clusterfuck that is 2020 are thousands of wildfires raging and destroying parts of my home state of California. Pictures from yesterday literally brought the word "Armageddon" to mind. It's raining ash. Our plants—everything outside, really—are covered with it, the skies are colors I haven't seen before, and the air reeks of smoke.

Yesterday, a woman from the US Census Bureau came to my door. Because of social distancing, we had to sit out on the patio to complete the survey and when we were done, both of us were covered in ash. We looked like the walking dead.

***

So many people are taking the edge off their pandemic anxiety by drinking. The response is real-Zoom Happy Hours are an official "thing" and retail sales of alcohol are up 32% compared to this time last year. (Brett is in wine sales. He and his bank account are quite happy with that number. His career is booming.) Yale School of Medicine experts warn against excessive drinking, stating it can increase susceptibility to and the severity of COVID-19 because it can compromise the immune system, raising the chances of getting Acute Respiratory Distress Syndrome (ARDS), a potentially fatal condition in which fluids can build in the lungs and a possible outcome of ending up on a ventilator. Add to that the ash and smoke of the wildfires irritating the lungs, which also increases the susceptibility to contracting COVID-19, and you've got one hell of a year. I am grateful that I am sober during all of this. I think about my friends and family who don't have the tools to weather these incredible storms. Stay safe. Stay present.

***

Today is the 19th anniversary of 9/11. It's a day of always remembering and reflection. It's one of those flashbulb memories where every single person who is old enough remembers exactly where they were that day. I was in the hallway of the Butte Building at Chico State University, waiting with a few other students for class. It was our second week of grad school. It was completely surreal. My daughter was completing her last year of college at the same time at the same campus and all I could think about was getting to her apartment to be with her.

Today, I also choose to reflect on what I have gained, rather than what I have lost or given up in my 14 months of sobriety. Sleep. Dignity. Self-respect. Integrity. Reconnection with a best friend. A deeper connection with another. New friends. A better relationship with my daughter. A better role model for my grandkids. A better marriage. My faith in God. Self-love. Growth. I am funnier. I listen more. This community. Meditation. Compassion. Love of nature.

Balance. Surrender. Prayer. Boundaries. Bird feeders. Forgiveness of myself and others. Love of books. Walking. Music. Dancing. Feeling. Laughing. Crying. Faith. Breathing. Knowing. Being present. Being completely silly. Being random. Being in awe. Being at peace. Just being. My truth. My soul.

***

Robert Brault wrote:

"Enjoy the little things in life because one day you'll look back and realize they were the big things." [57]

When I was drinking, appreciating the little things was fleeting, and often impossible for me. I just read an article about aging, which I am doing rather gracefully in sobriety. As well-adjusted people age, they naturally seek situations that lift their moods and enhance their well-being. It's good to know that wine, not my age, got in my way of my happiness. How flipping cool is that?

With that in mind, I thought I would share my September list of activities that support my intention to live with gratitude for all that I have, all that I am, allowing joy and love to fill my heart. Intentions are so important in alcohol-free living because they allow me to live in alignment with my core values and raise my emotional and physical energy. My list: restocking my s'mores box; creating my gratitude pumpkin (one for me and one for the grandkids, too); sending hand-written cards; watching the movie Mulan; re-watching the movies Up and Inside Out; putting up my Halloween decorations (one of my two favorite holidays); sewing at least six pineapple blocks on my new quilt; beginning "Trash Thursday" (picking up trash on my way back from my daily walk); ordering winter walking clothes/shoes; getting out my weighted blanket; and creating a photo book for our first grandson who turns 18 at the end of the month. What's on your list?

***

My friend Susan has been a tremendous supporter of my alcohol-free journey. As I mentioned before, she drinks one or two glasses of wine (slowly, I might add. Who ever heard of sipping wine?) and is perfectly fine with that. It's just who she is. I can't help but be envious sometimes. Yesterday I was in our local grocery store and everywhere I walked, boxes of wine were displayed throughout the entire store. Staring at me in the produce section were stacks of the sauvignon blanc brand I used to buy. On sale. For that split second, my mind and my mouth remembered that taste and smell of the first pour. I think how nice it would be to be a normal drinker, how nice it would be to have just one or two glasses. Most of my friends drink. Why can't I? But that fantasy dissipates into reality, and I'm reminded that even when I only drank occasionally, it was almost never one or two, and I would quickly descend down the rabbit hole. What comes to mind is the exhausting bargaining and promising behavior that results in me giving in and hating myself over and over and over again.

In her book *Drinking: A Love Story*, Caroline Knapp writes:

> "The struggle to control intake—modify it, cut it back, deploy a hundred different drinking strategies in the effort—is one of the most universal hallmarks of alcoholic behavior." [58] (If you haven't read this book, I highly recommend it.)

Last week, I came across a construction sign that spoke to me: ONE LANE ROAD AHEAD. We are all on different paths in our sober-minded journey, and some of you may be successful at moderation. That will never be me.

***

I was talking to a friend on Saturday who said she was spending so much time talking, texting, Zooming, and Marco-ing with her sober community that her husband thinks she is having an affair. I'm sure Paul has had that thought, too.

> "Recovery is a very selfish time for the individual going through it. It has to be that way. If you are not

putting your recovery first, then you are decreasing your chances of success." [59] —Katie Rietz

I know that going into my 15th month, Paul is extremely proud of me, and at the same time, he is wondering just how long I'm going to continue to spend tremendous amounts of my time and money on meetings, courses, and books. Answer: As long as it takes. He doesn't complain much, but I know he feels left out. I mean, it feels like I'm cheating on him sometimes. At this point in the book, y'all know way more about me than he does. It's not always easy for healthy, "normal" drinkers to understand addiction.

I am a social worker. Paul is a financial analyst. We are often on different planets. Our relationship is a balancing act where we are both aware that we need to make lots of adjustments to keep our relationship centered. It's hard work, for sure. Anything worth having is.

***

This one is tough for me to share. My sobriety has brought peace into my marriage, which was previously wrought with havoc and chaos. The emotional pain from the alcohol-fueled fights we had rivaled any physical pain I have experienced over my lifetime. For both of us. Heart. Breaking. Names were called, there was shoving, breaking of things. There was a lot of leaving, threats of divorce. It was just an overall shit show. There were times I absolutely had no recollection of the damage I had caused the night before. Sometimes our adult children were pulled into our mess. More. Hearts. Breaking. To summarize: I had turned into my mother.

Alcohol disrupts normal brain executive functioning and decision making. It is a major contributor to the occurrence of intimate partner violence, which is any behavior that causes sexual, physical, or psychological harm in a relationship. For either partner. It's nearly impossible to believe that our marriage didn't break. It didn't, because the only thing that was broken was the vicious, alcohol-fueled cycle of havoc and chaos.

There is still much work and healing to do. On both sides. We don't take for granted that the arguments we have these days involve such trivial, stupid things. Just yesterday, we both laughed when we argued about getting rid of some of the inherited moose décor in our cabin. I hate it. He loves it. FYI, there are no fucking moose near our cabin, or in the entire state of California, for that matter. It seriously looks like Cabela's threw up all over the place. A moose is most definitely NOT my spirit animal.

***

I enrolled in Laura McKowen's We Are the Luckiest: Sobriety in Living Color course near the time when COVID hit. One of the first assignments was to find something in my home that needed to be fixed and then fix it. I called to have my broken plantation shutters repaired and the feeling of satisfaction from doing that started a regular habit of fixing, decluttering, and straightening. I asked myself, do I need it? Do I love it? Has this item's moment passed? All of this is such a parallel process to my sober journey.

> "Our homes are an extension of who we are: what we do within the walls of our abodes shapes our mood, affects our productivity, and influences our outlook on life, making our life better." [60] —Jackie Ashton

I have developed all kinds of habits, including (but not limited to): making my bed every day; cleaning the kitchen before I go to bed (to be honest, Paul does this most of the time); going through my home/closet regularly to discard or donate; straightening my desk so that it's ready for class in the morning; making sure there is water in the Keurig for morning coffee; replacing worn towels and sheets; re-caulking the bathtubs; replacing burnt-out light bulbs; sharpening my colored pencils; replacing batteries in flameless candles—and the list goes on. My home has become a stress-free zone. My house is in order. So am I.

***

One of the biggest gifts of my sober life has been the ability to connect with other like-minded women and men in the virtual and social media world. It has been the silver lining of COVID because we have created many online resources as a result of the pandemic. I wish my mother, in her own struggle with alcohol, could have experienced this. My online connections have been one of the biggest reasons I went from countless day ones to day 433. Facebook, Instagram, Zoom, and Marco Polo—and yes, talking the old-fashioned way by telephone—have provided platforms where friendships are no longer limited by geography and time zones. I interact with people all over the world, all over the country and locally, with honesty and without judgment. If you haven't experienced this, you cannot comprehend the power of it. And when we turn those online friendships into real-life hugs, magic happens. This has happened several times in the past year, and there are plans for future meetups and visits. I got to welcome a sober sister's son from the Boston area to California, where he will attend his first year of college at UC Davis. Followed by a visit, lunch, and hugs from his mom shortly after. I love how these connections and friendships cross age barriers. I love the unconditional support when things get hard. I love knowing that other women and men understand the work it takes to get and stay sober. And I know my family wonders how it is possible to make such deep connections this way. We know.

***

More on Paul. No one suffered from my drinking more than my husband. Certainly, he contributed plenty to the issues in our marriage, but the out-of-control drinking that happened over the last ten years was and is my responsibility. I came across a term yesterday I had never heard before—"secondary drinking," which is the impact of repeatedly being exposed to your spouse's abusive drinking behaviors. That hit me right in the center of my heart. Secondary drinking describes what Paul went through with me. He had no significant issues with alcohol, so he didn't understand mine. He drinks an occasional beer or glass of wine. And there would be the intermittent holiday event where his consumption of bourbon with his four Irish sisters would result in professing his undying love for me repeatedly in the car on the way home. But that was the extent of it. My drinking was most definitely a family problem, and Paul was the receiver and the target of most of it. Like so many of you, my friends and colleagues didn't have a clue just how serious my drinking problem had become.

I asked Paul to describe some of his feelings about my drinking. "Are you social working me?" he asked. I said no, that I really wanted to know what he felt other than the apparent anger, disgust, and complete frustration my drinking caused. "Scared, anxious, missed the real me, humiliated, hurt, helpless, if-you-really-loved-me-you-would-quit, weak, hateful, alone, done." He threatened, he cried, he left, he came back, repeat. Paul talked about how reading *Alcohol Explained* and *This Naked Mind* turned his hurt and anger into compassion and understanding. It was then he became my biggest supporter.

Today, I honor him.

***

Matthew is my oldest child, but he is my second first child. The sister he never met died ten years before he was born. I guess you would say he's my rainbow baby.

Matt is the hardest child for me to talk about because although he has been the least affected by my drinking, he has been the most affected by divorce. At six, I thought it was the right thing to move him away from his perfectly good father to live closer to my husband's children. I more than willingly spent the next ten years driving an hour to meet his dad at the same half-way point, The Nut Tree in Vacaville, where a shit-load of divorced parents met on Sunday nights to exchange children with their exes. (We became an odd family of sorts, watching each other's kids grow up.)

Matt ended up moving back in with his father in his sophomore year of high school. That broke my heart. But I knew in that same heart, it was the right decision.

If you asked Matt if I ever had a drinking problem, he would probably say "no," although—just like his brother—I put him in a position where he felt he needed to defend me from his stepfather at a wedding where I drank too much. Police responded to the hotel. Thank God, one of my daughter's friends is a detective and talked the officer out of arresting Matt. He never once held this incident against me.

Matthew is a quiet, caring, sensitive father of three. He has a great sense of humor and can dance like his paternal grandfather. He is a brilliant writer of rap lyrics. Our love for writing has been a surprising and cherished connection between the two of us. After reading a draft of this book, he wrote these words:

Went from full of life, was the life of the party
To hardly remembering, denial, then saying sorry
Image of yourself is blurry, looking pretty hazy
Woke up like nothing went wrong, the night went amazing
Being told what you did, footsteps being retraced
If you don't remember it, then it never really happened
No need to pay for the consequences of your actions
Everything's not so clear, things don't seem as they appear
Who's judging who? When you're staring in the mirror
Constantly misdirected by your own misconceptions
Ducking and deflecting questions about personal reflections
We go through phases of life, throughout the different stages
Times can be rough, so adapt and make the changes
Sometimes the word "hope" just isn't enough
So we need the strength and knowledge to rise above
Free, yet I'm in prison, trapped in mental captivity
When darkness surrounds you, you'll need the light to see
Getting wasted, that's a waste of time, time is hard to find
There's no way to rewind it, so you'll have to change your mind
The bottle has got you off balance, feeling a bit tipsy
So can I lean on you, your dependability is iffy
Is this what you wanted and expected from your life?
Faithful to the drink, need to revive to survive
Your lack of vision has got you missing, lifeless drifting
Suffering from the life you are not living, drinking is so addicting

Alcohol has one intent, that to leave you with nothing left
Soul ripped from your chest, hope you can accept that debt
So remember to tip … pour it out, not another drop
Take control and flip the script, don't lose that grip
The line in the sand has been drawn, which way will you respond?
Tell me, which side of alcohol are you on?

***

The other night, I met up with a few new sober friends at a local restaurant. One of them asked if it was hard for me to attend social events where everyone was drinking, because it was still difficult for her. I'm not big on giving advice. I truly believe all our paths are different. I know for me, I have fiercely and selfishly protected my sobriety at all costs. That includes being extremely discriminating about what social events I show up at, and I still make sure I use my own transportation so I can leave whenever I want. I say, "No, thank you." A lot. This is especially true when it comes to people and places where I just don't feel like I fit in.

COVID has been a nightmare for so many people, but it has given me permission to stay home from events I might have felt obligated to attend. I'm just venturing out socially after a year, and I noticed something about myself at tonight's meetup. It's still awkward socializing without a glass of sauvignon blanc in my hand. I wonder if I'm talking too much or not listening enough. I feel vulnerable, and at the same time, it feels so cool. Who knew you could have so much fun without alcohol? I feel a bit like a social virgin. I mean, I haven't really experienced adult social life without the lubricating effect of alcohol to get me through for years. I used to feel sorry for people who don't drink. Does that make any sense?

I love this meme:

"1. Going to bed early.
2. Not leaving my house.
3. Not going to a party.
My childhood punishments have become my adult goals." [61]

In doing this work I discovered I have a large, introverted side to my personality. Introversion is a trait that is defined as more of a focus on the internal thoughts and feelings than on external stimulation. This was so surprising to me. I have always thought of myself as an extrovert. I'm sure that if you asked most anyone, they would say I am a social butterfly. I absolutely love people. All kinds of people. I have a serious sense of humor. I don't mind getting up in front of large groups to teach or give presentations. I'm not shy. I can hang with people I have never met before.

It's so clear to me now that I am a combination of both. Looking back, I usually drank when I was around large groups. Big gatherings like the annual family picnic made me super-anxious. I have realized that my uncomfortableness in crowds has been the impetus for so much of my over-drinking. I don't care for wedding and baby showers. Simply put, I suck at small talk. I often engaged in "pre-drinking" just to get through an event, or I would down a couple glasses of wine upon arrival. I remember being at my daughter's wedding where there were over 200 people, many of them I hadn't seen in years. Not being able to pay attention to them individually filled me with anxiety. I felt like Gumby.

I know that having all my family over was a source of anxiety for me. I also know now that drinking alcohol is like putting jet fuel on anxiety. Some of these events were the site of some less than proud drinking behavior. And this only worked to validate the negative opinions some family members have of me.

I love my family and friends so much, but after their visits, I am depleted. I need to recharge in my bedroom or watch mindless shows on TV. I also need a lot of "me time" after a day of teaching when I feel like a balloon that someone just let the air out of.

I am still social, but in different ways. I have discovered my love for one-on-one meetups. Would I like to go for a walk and talk? Sure. Coffee at Starbucks? I'm there. How about a trip to the nursery and lunch? I would love to. Wanna set up a Zoom call? What time and when?

I choose the larger gatherings I want to attend, and I always have an exit plan. I drive my own car. Amanda Ward and Jardine Libaire (*The Sober Lush*) call this "The Vanish":

> "She took a deep breath. And then she vanished— only to reappear in her pajamas, safe and warm, where she belonged, in bed." [62]

I so love that …

***

It turns out that being needy is a good thing. All my life I received the message that expressing my needs is selfish, and it was highly discouraged. I don't think, until now, I have ever been able to communicate what I need to anyone. This certainly contributed to my drinking. How frustrating it must have been for my husband, who has often thrown up his hands and screamed at me: "What the fuck do you want, Peggi?" or "You don't even know what you need!" I have no problem expressing my needs now. (Right, Paul?)

I cannot expect my husband or anyone I have a relationship with to be a mind reader. Something that may seem obvious to me may not be obvious to them. In the new world order, I now express my needs all over the place. "I need for you and Brett to be civil with each other." (Of course.) "I need to do something different this year for Thanksgiving. Do you mind if we go to my brother's house in Arizona instead of your sister's?" (Yes, I think that's a great idea. I love Jerry.) "We need to purge and replace the fucking moose furniture at the cabin." (Well, that may be a bit more challenging …) Dr. Jenev Caddell writes:

> "You have wired in biological needs for a safe and secure emotional connection, no matter who you are. Add to those wired in biological needs, a history of maybe not having all of your needs met (let's face it, not everyone had a perfect childhood), and those needs may be stronger. We need stuff from our partners. We need to

feel valuable, important, understood, seen, heard and appreciated." [63]

P.S. I need all of you.

***

Today is a harder share than most. I woke up feeling like I have a hangover and I am super-weepy. I went to my first large social gathering in over 14 months last night. It was my friend Susan's birthday.

Yesterday, I had the best time picking out all the stuff I needed to make one of my famous charcuterie trays. It was a colossal hit. I had so much fun picking out Susan's gifts. I seriously LOVE and adore her family and friends. So much. I could even share my sobriety story with a couple of friends who appeared very interested in my alcohol-free journey. I did wince when the word "alcoholic" was tossed into the conversation, but I love the person who said it, and felt comfortable to explain my feelings about the term. This friend ended up telling me about her own daughter's struggles with alcohol. I shared some of my resources and she was so grateful.

So, why did I feel so socially uncomfortable? I didn't feel shy; I didn't lack self-confidence. I just felt awkward. I thought to myself, "Why can't I party like everyone else?"

Megan Rogers, LCSW seemed to be inside my head when she wrote this:

> "What I uncovered is that a) my love of planning was actually just that. It was never the actual party or event that I enjoyed. Because b) in reality, I felt awkward and uncomfortable around people unless they were my closest people, actually. And even as a kid, I felt like I never fit in. This is one of the biggest ways that alcohol hooked me two decades ago, BECAUSE c) I thought I was an extrovert but really, I was just drunk and I'm actually an introvert and d) alcohol masked this, was a

quick and easy way for me to feel comfortable and at ease with people and not socially anxious. Crap!" [64]

Ahhh, it's all a process of finding out who I really am, right? Thank you for listening.

***

I will never stop being grateful for all the time that has been added to my life since I stopped drinking. I continue to be in awe of just how much I can accomplish/notice/take in now that I am present every day. These are some of my favorite things I have done, received, or observed recently that have brought joy to myself and others: peppermint eucalyptus shower bombs; buying a new bathmat at TJ Max (there's nothing like a beautiful bargain to lift your spirits); petting and giving treats to neighborhood dogs (I received a card from a neighborhood dog's owner addressed as "Maggie's favorite human"); buying Rae Dunn grocery list note pads for $2.50 instead of writing on the back of anything (buying anything Rae Dunn at TJ Max or Home Goods makes me happy); buying myself flowers; making a care package for my friend's son for his first day in his college dorm; getting transparent post-it note pads from a friend (you have to get some!); taking my daughter and her family out to dinner to introduce them to my maid of honor at my wedding; waving to my favorite elderly couple sunning in their wheelchairs on my morning walk (I learned that the woman's name is Anna and she blows me kisses now); not recognizing a colleague/friend/neighbor who, during COVID, has lost over 60 pounds (go, Amy!); having a sober sister drop in for lunch (thank you, Julie); making a birthday charcuterie tray; getting out my Halloween decorations (and not finding empty wine bottles); and writing a special letter to our first grandson who turns 18 today (happy birthday, Luke). Ah, life is good.

***

I sat down on my bed this morning, ready to write today's post, and I spilled a whole cup of Kona coffee all over my damn self, the quilt, blanket, sheets, and mattress pad. It went everywhere except on the carpet. Something like this would have ruined my day pre-AF, but all I could think about as I stripped down the bedding was how happy I was that it wasn't wine I'd spilled, like so many times in the past. I was grateful it didn't get on the carpet. And because the coffee got on almost everything, tonight I will climb into bed with clean, fresh bedding enhanced by lavender and sea salt spray. And I found this little gem of a story that made this experience even more meaningful:

> "You are holding a cup of coffee when someone comes along and bumps into you or shakes your arm making you spill your coffee. 'Why did you spill the coffee?' 'Well, because someone bumped into me, of course!' Wrong answer. You spilled the coffee because there was coffee in your cup. Had there been tea [or wine] in the cup you would have spilled tea [or wine]. Whatever is in the cup will spill out. When life comes along and shakes you (which WILL happen), whatever is inside you will come out. It's easy to fake it until you get rattled. So, we have to ask ourselves, 'What's in my cup?' When life gets tough, what spills over?" [65] —Author unknown

***

Yesterday, I had a virtual classroom experience from hell. I was a facilitator in a planning session and my director was in the meeting. I facilitated a group who was less than enthusiastic about being in the meeting; the purpose was to improve outcomes for children and families in the child welfare system. On top of that, I got kicked out of Zoom and it took me about ten excruciating minutes to get back into the meeting.

Q: What does my shittiest COVID workday have to do with sobriety?

A: I had this almost insatiable urge to apologize to my boss for what happened. I stopped writing the email and asked myself why I felt the need to apologize for something over which I had absolutely no control.

In sobriety, I am learning that some things literally have nothing to do with me. I deleted the email. If I did nothing wrong, why would I want people to think I did? My director reiterated this in our debriefing meeting. She described the session as "pretty rough" and complimented me on the way I hung in there and made it through.

In contrast, raging at my husband this morning because our internet went down in our condo three hours away from the cabin (where he was), yet fully expecting him to do something about it, is a completely different story, was definitely my bad, and called for a rather strong apology from me.

**

During my morning walk, and during many, many walks this year, I think about one other family member who had to be so affected by my drinking—our Schnauzer, Rex. I don't think I could ever describe the depth of love I had (have) for that little guy. Our grandkids grew up with him. He loved everyone. He patiently let the kids dress him up in all kinds of costumes, drag him on walks around the house, knowing he would be rewarded by spilled cheerios and French fries.

Rex was a witness to my worst drinking years.

That means he had to endure many of the fights Paul and I had over, or that were caused by, alcohol. I know that so many times he watched what was going on and it would scare him. He would tremble and run under the bed. I don't know how many times Paul and I would stop arguing to tell him, "Rex, we're okay, it's okay." Both of us would feel like shit when we saw what our arguing was doing to him.

When humans argue, dogs don't understand what's happening and they feel helpless. Dogs are much like children in their reaction to adult behavior. They actually get filled with the stress hormone cortisol, just as we do.

ıl loved Rex so much that I sometimes think he stayed with
ɔause he couldn't bear to live without him. When we had to
put Rex down last year, I had never seen my husband cry like that.
Ever. In 34 years. Shit, I'm bawling, just writing this. Anyway, buddy,
I hope you are running with the big dogs now and can see from that
rainbow bridge that things are pretty good. Always in our hearts.

***

The other day, I came across an album with memorabilia from
the dance, aerobics, theater, and art studio I owned and directed in
the 1990s called Heart and Sole and later, when I added the non-
profit Colusa County Performing Arts. We put on recitals, The
Nutcracker, art exhibits, Haunted Houses, and various theater
productions in partnership with the local school district and
community college. Kids who didn't want to dance or act had the
opportunity to learn lighting and set design. I also had a side gig
choreographing the high school show choir, marching band and
flag team.

I had forgotten what a big deal the dance studio was because I
was too busy being full of self-loathing for what I had become.

This is why I am so committed to staying on this side of alcohol.
No more living small. I am that creative person once again. I am
who I was meant to be all along.

***

At the core of all curricula I teach to social workers is Safety
Organized Practice (SOP). This team-based practice is grounded in
the belief that parents and caretakers are experts on their own
families, are capable of change, and (with support) are able to
identify the behavior changes they need to make to keep their

children safe. In its simplest form, SOP asks three questions: What
are we worried about? What is working well? What are the next
steps we need to take? The answers to those questions create
customized safety plans for each individual family.

I noticed that this practice is so parallel to the work I have been
doing on my sobriety journey. For almost 15 months, I have been

asking myself the same questions in one form or another. The answers have propelled me forward in creating my own unique plan of alcohol-free living. For all of us seeking sobriety, the answers are different, depending on our individual strengths, needs, and life experiences. There is no "one size fits all" for any of us on our path to recovery. That's why it's so important to try many approaches and to see what truly works for you. There is so much out there. Every one of us can make changes in our lives. We just have to take that first step.

***

For many of you, it seems like one of your challenges to get and/or stay sober is having a partner who either drinks or encourages you to drink again, and/or expresses some sort of sadness/disappointment that they have lost their "fun drinking buddy." I can appreciate the challenge that might be.

That isn't my experience. For me, there is always that thought in the back of my mind that picking up a glass of wine would mean losing the relationship with my daughter I have worked so hard to rebuild, and my marriage would most likely be over. Most of the time, I consider my daughter's and my husband's intervention to be a blessing. But occasionally, the fleeting thought comes across my mind that I want to KNOW I would choose not to drink even if I didn't have those threats hanging over me. At 450 days, I have almost no desire to drink now or ever again. I do have the rare fantasy of a glass of champagne at a wedding, or that first taste of sauvignon blanc, but they are fleeting thoughts. I hope I would have made the decision to stop drinking on my own, but I will never know the answer to that. I do know that, at the time of my last drink, I didn't love myself enough to quit, but I did love my daughter.

What does matter is that I know I wouldn't be writing this post if Lindsay and Paul hadn't stepped in. I shudder to think where I would be instead. I'm humbled by that thought.

***

I was putting on my makeup this morning and it reminded me of my drinking days when it would take twice as long to apply it because I often felt like total crap and my hands would be shaking uncontrollably. Putting in my contacts could be more than challenging as well. I rarely went out of the house without makeup or doing my hair, because I had convinced myself it would keep people from figuring out I had been drinking the night before. Hope sprang eternal.

I would put on concealer, primer, foundation, powder, blush, eyeshadow. (Haha … at 68, I need it ALL!) Then I would put on my eyeliner and my shaking hands would cause the liner to go on crooked or, even worse, shoot across my eyelid, completely missing its intended destination altogether, making me a look-alike for Cruella de Vil And I would have to start all over again.

It shocks Paul that I often go out of the house now with no makeup at all. And I do it with confidence. Ah, the perks and freedoms of an alcohol-free life.

***

I spent the last two days at our cabin with my new sober friend Stacy. This experience prompted me to reflect on the monumental shift in my friendships and relationships during my 10,848 hours (but who's counting?) of alcohol-free living. Some of those shifts have left me with a myriad of emotions, sometimes sad, sometimes hurt, and sometimes relieved. In doing this work, I'm learning what I truly want out of life and the people I want in it. Some didn't make the cut, and that's okay.

I have let some friendships go, reconnected, moved to deeper, more meaningful friendships with others, and have been able to let so many beautiful, new, like-minded people into my life. I have made myself vulnerable by reaching out to people I resonate with and want to get to know better. By putting myself out there, I have found my voice and, hopefully, have inspired others to do the same. Believe me, it is so worth the risk. PS: Our dinner at Highlands Ranch Resort in Mineral was one of the best I have had. The hot beignets with chocolate sauce were to die for!

***

Other than family, I don't think that I have had a house guest since I stopped drinking in July 2019. Oh wait, I had one overnight guest, a colleague/friend who came to collaborate on some curricula we were updating.

When Stacy and I made plans to spend a couple days here at the cabin, I panicked a bit. I have become fiercely protective of my morning routine because my sobriety depends on structure. Paul is fully aware of this and gives me all the space I need.

I had that divided mind that Jenn Kautsch talks about. I wanted Stacy to feel at home and comfortable, and I also needed my routine that has kept me on my sober path for almost 15 months. I talked with Stacy, told her what I needed, and she was totally supportive. The old me would have ceded to "people pleasing" and I probably would have never brought it up. And then I would have been full of resentment.

Alicia Gilbert from Soberish writes:

> "Morning routines are the 'in' thing in health and wellness right now, but it's honestly not without reason. For the vast majority of us, early sobriety is a confusing, frustrating time. Our brains love patterns and habit. [Morning routines] will keep you busy, focused on making positive changes and help you heal from the damage alcohol has done on your mental and physical well-being." [66]

My current morning routine: I get up around 5:00 am (I consistently go to bed between 9:00 and 10:00 pm), drink water, have my Kona coffee, say my Surrender Novena prayers, write, do homework on any class I am currently enrolled in, review training notes if I am teaching that day, go on a walk, shower, get ready by listening to my favorite music, and finish with a light breakfast.

Do whatever works for you.

***

A couple days ago, I had what I would describe as a complete food overdose. I was so proud of myself for going out to dinner Monday night and eating only two of those five heavenly beignets I had ordered for dessert with Stacy. (Note that during my drinking days, I rarely—and I mean rarely—ordered dessert at a restaurant, choosing instead to drink my dessert.) Anyway, the next day, I proceeded to eat cinnamon-sugar toast, the rest of the beignets (with chocolate sauce), several Nips peanut butter hard candy, cheese, TWO servings of chicken cordon blue (Paul decided not to drive up to the cabin that day and I had cooked both, so I couldn't waste it, right?), leftover Spanish rice and a mini-ice cream cone (size matters, you know). Yesterday, I woke up with what had to have been a major sugar hangover. Ugh. To say my wedding ring was tight was an understatement.

Grateful for the lessons learned in my alcohol-free journey and *Atomic Habits*, I chose not to beat myself up or develop a case of the "fuck-its." I didn't weigh myself (usually a daily thing for me) and considered Tuesday to be an outlier in my normal routine. I stayed calm. It's just food. Whatever I do today is something I am leaving behind.

***

There was a time when coming to my local grocery store was more important than coming home. As soon as I was done with teaching I would think, "Is there wine at home? Do I need to stop and buy some?" Nugget Market became an integral part of my daily routine. On the weekends, I would come up with every excuse in the book to go to the store. I appreciated that it had at least a dozen checkout stands so I could pick a different one, and hopefully a different checker, each day.

Only people with alcohol issues would even think about shit like that. I mentioned before that sometimes I would buy a greeting card or a wine gift bag so the checker would think I was buying the wine for someone else. WTF? Pure craziness. Paul asked me the other day why I have at least 30 almost-as-pricey-as-wine gift bags stacked in the cabinet. I need to toss or donate them. They are really one of the last visual reminders of the life I have left behind.

Now, I find every excuse in the book NOT to go grocery shopping. Last week, I went five entire days without going to the store. A personal best! And guess what? Instead of falling asleep on the couch with all that wine running through my veins, my evenings got so much bigger. I come home to a place where I can catch up with a friend, study a curriculum, write, watch TV (and remember what I watched), join an online recovery meeting, and have actual conversations with my husband (when he has his hearing aids in). What's not to love?

∗∗∗

I am currently teaching a six-part series on Child and Family Team Meeting Facilitation, and we talk a lot about dealing with the anxiety and stress of getting up and essentially performing in front of a group of people. This had me reflecting on how I ever got up after a night of drinking to teach or present. The hangxiety I experienced following a night of drinking was almost paralyzing.

> "The physical responses to being hungover—dehydration, nausea, rapid heartbeat—are so similar to anxiety, these symptoms can trigger anxiety attacks" [67] —Tabitha Vidaurri

Add to that the shame and anxiety I felt after a night where I blacked out. Paul wouldn't be talking to me or he might have left for the hundredth time. What a perfect storm. No! What a perfect shit-storm.

I became so convinced that no matter how many hours I spent studying and preparing, my students and my colleagues could see right through me and see that I was a fraud. It was pure torture.

I know that:

> "A certain amount of anxiety is useful, even indispensable. Anxiety can be helpful … and provide the extra mental charge to think through choices. Getting rid of all traces of anxiety would be like successfully dismantling your house's security system." [68] —Ken Eisold

My drinking made it impossible to tell the difference between good anxiety and bad. These days, I welcome that anxiety. It keeps me prepared, focused, motivated, present, and excited about life. I am fully living my passion as a teacher of social work. And so very grateful.

***

During these 15 months of sobriety, I have increasingly been buying books like there is an apocalypse coming. When someone reads or quotes a passage that resonates with me, I order the book. If someone makes a recommendation, I buy the book. Damn you, Amazon! I bought several books twice. I am out of control. (Anyone out there know a support group for bookaholics?) It feels a bit like the almost painful memories of my frenzied participation in the total consumer anarchy of Cabbage Patch Dolls and Beanie Babies. Guess how old I am? How about those pet rocks? Now how old am I? I am shamefully admitting I was one of THOSE mothers. Now, I am not comparing toys with books, just the behavior. I have always adored books. Always. Currently, I have at least 20 books I haven't read yet and I am coming clean with all of you so that maybe, just maybe, it will motivate me to hit the pause button before I hit "place order."

On the flip side, when it comes to choosing something new to read, no matter what mood I am in, I can "shop" on my shelves.

***

By being totally present, I have learned that I can't make time go by more quickly and I can't stop it from passing. Each morning when I wake up, after reciting my Surrender Novena, I ask myself: "What is one thing I can do today that will bring me closer to my goals? What lesson will I learn from my action or inaction? What is something I can do today that my future self will be thankful for, proud of?"

I love this quote from The Joy Blog:

> "It may be hard to take it one day at a time when you are having your cravings. Maybe you could take it ten minutes at a time. Choose sobriety for the next ten

minutes. Then when those ten minutes end, you can choose again what you're going to do with the next ten minutes after that. Suddenly you made it through an hour, then half a day, then a full week, then a month. All of that combines to a year, and then a lifetime." [69]

I know that my future can only be shaped by the things I do 24 hours at a time. Every day, I treat sobriety as if my life depends on it. Because it does. Whenever I am in doubt, whenever the thought crosses my mind that having a glass of wine would be wonderful again, I think about my last drink and how it almost cost me everything.

***

We have an activity in one of our social work trainings where we ask students to imagine and describe what it might feel like to move from one location to a completely new one. We do this to encourage the development of empathy and compassion for what it feels like for our child welfare parents to make challenging behavioral changes in their lives. This had me thinking how packing up and moving to a new location is so parallel to my alcohol-free journey. At first, both can leave you feeling lonely, unsettled, unsure, afraid, and ungrounded. Both require getting used to living in an entirely new community. I experienced this when we moved to West Sacramento from our home in Colusa where we lived and raised our children for over 30 years.

My co-workers hosted a retirement party that ended with hugs and tears and promises to stay in touch. That happened for a while, but what bound us together no longer existed and almost all those friendships are gone or have been reduced to Facebook, Instagram, and/or Christmas cards.

Sobriety can affect friendships in the same way. Some of my friends and family don't fit in or don't want to fit in with my alcohol-free lifestyle. Some are not interested in knowing the work it took to get here. A few hung in there with me and became my biggest cheerleaders, and we now enjoy a deeper, more meaningful connection. Some friends and family walked away when I needed support the most and, as much as that hurt, I know they aren't the people I need to have in my life, at least for now. Transitions are hard. It can be a positive thing, but you're leaving behind the world you knew and must start over in many areas of life. The upside is that sobriety has freed me to reach out and form new relationships. And that has been one of sobriety's biggest gifts.

***

On October 15, 2019, I wrote my first reason-I-am-grateful-to-be-AF post. I was 94 days into my sober-minded journey, two days before I arrived at the Sober Sis Retreat in Fort Worth. I didn't know that I would still be writing them 365 days later. I had no idea that the posts and all of you would become such an integral, non-negotiable part of my daily sobriety routine. I had originally committed myself to writing them for 100 days. It turned out to be 366. Writing has allowed me to grow in my mind, body, and soul in ways I never thought were possible for me. What started out as an accountability exercise became much bigger than me. Words started pouring out of me at an indescribable rate. Yes, there were days I had no idea what to write and after reciting my surrender prayer, the words would come. Some days I would hear a gentle voice telling me, "Write about this today." I listened.

On October 15, 2020, I wrote my last daily post so that I could focus my efforts on writing this book. I switched to weekly posts each Monday.

Being sober has allowed me to receive and hear the invitations sent to me by God and the Universe. It has allowed me to be open to all the possibilities that living alcohol free offers. And, of course, Sevens see the possibilities in everything (when they are sober). I am accepting the very loud invitation to explore what is next for me.

***

I really must share how hard it was to wake up last Friday and not post after doing it every single day for an entire year. Even though I am replacing the time with writing my book, I felt sad, anxious, and out of sorts. I guess it's the growing pains of taking on something new and leaving some of the familiar. Routine has been such a foundational piece of my sobriety. I have also learned that being right outside my comfort zone is the optimum way I learn. I was surprised at my mix of emotions.

Along with this change, I'm feeling the powerful pull to go public with my story. It has been comfortable and safe for me to be brave in the recovery community, but the "invitation" to share my story with the outside world grows stronger every day. I have big worries. How will this affect my career, my family, especially my daughter? In the end, my need to be authentic and to be of service to others is winning out. I am so completely proud of what I have been able to accomplish over the last 15 months and how my life has changed for the better. There will be people who will judge me. That's okay. This is who I am now. Candidly sharing my successes and struggles with you has been life altering. I want that same thing for others who have no idea how amazing life can be on this side of alcohol. I plan to share my story on my Instagram account next Sunday.

Another quote from one of my favorite humans across the pond, Louise: "Stepping off a cliff is having the belief that my wings are actually going to work."

***

On October 19, 2019, I was at the Sober Sis retreat in Fort Worth, Texas. I was 99 days alcohol free. Jenn Kautsch asked all the attendees to write a note to ourselves as if one year had passed, intending to mail them out on this year's October 19. I had absolutely no memory of what I wrote. I remember being uncomfortable doing it, not really knowing what to write. I just received this in the mail. I am completely humbled by the words I don't remember writing:

> Dear Peggi:
> One year from now I want to be 465 days AF. I want to be sharing my life experiences with others who want to go on this alcohol-free journey. I also want to share this with child welfare moms and dads who find themselves in a bad relationship with alcohol. I want to inspire others. Congratulations for accomplishing all of this!

How cool is this?

I took the giant leap yesterday. After talking to my director and my daughter, I posted about my sobriety journey on Instagram for the entire world to see. Truth be told, I have some feelings of buyer's remorse. I wouldn't want to walk it back; it's just how I am feeling right now—vulnerable.

***

My friend Jeff told his sobriety story last week, and it literally rocked me to my core. He talked about his adult daughter finding him passed out in his truck on Super Bowl day. "I bought a two-hour buzz. I can't get rid of the memory I gave my daughter seeing her dad like that." I cried listening to him. His was the plot to my story, to so many of our stories.

Which brings us to last Saturday when my daughter picked up the kids after a sleepover. She announced that she and Jason are taking Paul and me to Hawaii next year for Spring Break. I immediately began leaking tears. Lots of them. Pouring. "Mom, why are you crying?" I'm welling up again, just writing this. "Lindsay, these are happy tears. I'm just so grateful. For everything."

Lindsay could have told me she was taking me anywhere and it would have meant the same thing. I have my daughter back. The ask meant so much more than the destination.

And to quote Jeff again, who nailed it with this: "I can't take back the memory that I gave to my kids, but I changed the ending." Yes, my friend, we certainly did.

***

I love how sobriety has made me a better friend. To existing friends, new friends, and ones I have yet to meet. Some of my friends do life the way I do, some do it differently. And if I have learned anything in my 68 years, it's that the world needs diversity, the strength of multiple persons, to make it go around. My friends and I do life based on honesty, truth, vulnerability, and compassion; things I was often incapable of being when I was drinking. Just recently, a best friend of mine who was having a really rough time asked me to come over, and because I no longer drink, I could come right over and be totally present for her. That felt good.

I am more intentional with friendships. We set up dates for phone calls or video chats, and when we can't, we text or message to check in with each other. We accommodate for all the different time zones. We make actual plans to meet, to go on walks, go shopping, have dinner. I find I am putting the same effort into friendships as I do into sobriety. Both are precious to me. Of course, there is still spontaneity, but I make sure that I connect with my friends in a more meaningful and purposeful way. The return on investment is exponential.

My friends make me brave.

"I am a good friend to my friends, and they to me. Without them, there would be nothing to say to you today because I would be a cardboard cutout. But I call them on the phone, and I meet them for lunch. I show up. I listen. I laugh." [70] —Anna Quindlen

***

It's not about having a low bottom, a rock bottom, a hangover, or a blackout. If that were true, I would have quit drinking long before I did. It was that internal struggle of wanting to be sober more than I wanted to drink. It's how I felt on the inside with all the lies that took me so far from my true self, I didn't recognize the person staring back at me in the mirror. Now I do. And I love her again.

On my walk today, I came across a discarded empty wine bottle. I see lots of empty bottles on my walks. I used to be so judgmental of the person who threw it there. Now, I wonder if there is a story behind the bottle that might be like mine. Now I pray, if she or he reaches out, there will be someone there to listen like there was for me.

***

I was invited to share my sobriety story with a group of women last Thursday. I was so completely honored to be asked. Even though

I have been sharing my story for over a year through my writing, telling it in this setting was so cathartic and meaningful for me. My eyes were leaking several times during the telling and I appreciated the "that was me, too" comments at the end.

I am currently reading the book *Group*, by Christie Tate, who writes about her eating disorder which parallels alcohol abuse.

> "Holding on to secrets is a way to hold shame that doesn't belong to you ... the defining feature of my eating [drinking] disorder was secrecy." [71]

When I heard that voice, that tap on my shoulder, that I needed to go public, I jumped in with my whole mind, body, and soul. In telling my story, including the defining incident that finally led me to stop drinking, my prayer is that my words can be a changing, or sustaining, or resonating moment for someone. I still get a hitch in my breathing when I see a comment from a colleague or a friend who didn't know I was carrying such a secret. Most comments are supportive. "Oh, my gosh! I love this!!! You never cease to amaze me." "Love ya, friend! Keep up the good work." "I'm so proud of you! And it's amazing that you're going to help so many other people. Love u, lady!"

***

I want people to understand how drinking affected my life and the lives of people that I love. I believe that when I share my story

and you share yours, we change attitudes, views, and perceptions of alcohol abuse. We learn from our mistakes, but we also make some great choices in sobriety. We put humanity into recovery. And I am available to others in a way I have never been available before. I am learning how to truly live this sober life of mine.

***

Sober milestones are starting to go by without notice. Counting days had been such an integral part of my sobriety that it surprises me when I miss "day count" milestones and yet, it made me smile inside.

Maybe this one passed by because my two sets of twin grandkids were here for a sleepover. I was preoccupied—in awe, really, of how four children could blanket our condo in toys and leave foot and handprints on every single open space of our hardwood floors. Extremely talented kids. They definitely take after me.

I know that counting days has become less and less critical; I find myself paying attention to bigger milestones. Counting has become less of an obsession and more of an observation. Because I post weekly, I just add seven days to last week's post.

What I know is that I'm not the same person I was 523 days ago.

Counting was indispensable in my early days of sobriety—a potent motivator to get me through some really fucking difficult and lonely times when the only thing going right that day was that I didn't pick up a drink. As I stacked up the days, I couldn't help but feel a sense of accomplishment.

I know that for some people, counting can be a reminder of the enormity of quitting for good. And for those who do pick up a drink after a period of sobriety, it's so important to know that all that growth is still there. It hasn't gone away. You are still moving in the direction of becoming your most authentic self.

***

I was at the cabin last weekend; I got up at my usual 5:00 am and found my son-in-law Jason in the kitchen having coffee. I asked him what he was doing up so early and he said he has made a habit of getting up at about five to have some time for himself. By doing that, he says, he feels more prepared and awake for the day, he has more patience with the kids, and his days go significantly better.

Jason has been witness to many of my ugly drinking scenes, which started about the time he and Lindsay began dating over ten years ago. Sometimes I wonder how he still wants to be around me. He is an amazing, caring human, husband, and father to two sets of twins. I would have picked him out for Lindsay because he complements her in so many ways. I watch them sometimes and I see how well they fit together and make such a great team.

Jason did something that morning that made me know I had climbed higher on my mountain. He asked how my sobriety was going, asked if I missed drinking, asked if it bothered me when other people drink, asked if all those AF drinks I have make me ever want the real thing. It was an easy, interactive conversation. I told him all about my book, my Facebook page, my recent podcast interview, the things I have done and plan to do to maintain being alcohol free. He was interested in all of it. I cannot tell you how comfortable I felt talking to him. It was like the elephant had finally left the room.

This was such a beautiful conversation not only because it brought Jason and me closer, but also because I know that much of our conversation will be relayed to my daughter, who shows her love and support for my sobriety in many ways, but has a harder time talking face-to-face about it. When I shared this with my friend Louise, she offered this: "So often in recovery we are provided with opportunities to have conversations, to make amends without forcing them or driving the timeline. They appear soft and gently when we are ready to speak and to be heard."

I drove home with a very full heart.

***

Around this time last year, I finished Laura McKowen's book *We Are the Luckiest,* and although her book has had such a profound impact on my life, I really didn't understand the meaning of the title of her book. I had been sober for almost seven months. I certainly didn't consider myself lucky that I was one of THOSE people who couldn't drink like a normal person.

Now, at almost 19 months sober, I get it. I actually feel sorry for people who have never had a drinking problem because many of them haven't been inspired or motivated to do the work I have done and continue to do—to become my most authentic self and to strive to be the best person possible. To be the best mother, grandmother, wife, teacher, writer, and friend.

Words and concepts like mindfulness, transformation, meditation, self-love, movement, truth, curiosity, moving-through-the-pain, surrender, self-compassion, peace, wholeness, and breathing are integrated into my very being and everyday practice.

I get it now. We ARE the luckiest.

***

On the Monday morning after the Super Bowl (if you can call it that), my son Brett called me to say he was hungover. He is 37, so the experience is a completely normal and socially acceptable one to him and his friends. There was the usual joking and recounting of the events of the previous evening. In the background, there was the affirming laughter of his adorable girlfriend.

About five minutes into the conversation, Brett asked me if I would ever drink again.

Nope.

Drinking violated every core value I had—integrity, growth, freedom, curiosity, justice, and humor. (Well, I'm pretty sure I was still quite funny.)

With alcohol, I lied, blacked out, woke up feeling like total shit on many days for the last several years, repeatedly broke promises to myself and others. I came very, very close to losing everything I loved.

So, no, Brett, I have no plans to pick up that glass again. I'm sure I don't want to be remembered as that "poor lady we lost to alcohol."

I am doing things I never thought possible. My relationships with family, friends, and colleagues feel brand-new. I take care of myself. I feel worthy. I am more. I am amazing. And I am even more hilarious than ever.

***

Valentine's Day is next Sunday. It's a Hallmark holiday that can feel forced and inherent with single shaming. A day that can remind you of not being in a relationship or being in a bad or mediocre one. It certainly can be the source of feeling lonely or sad, triggering a response to think about picking up that drink.

When I was first married to Sonny and enrolled in college, we worked at Cattlemen's Steak House where people would wait up to two hours to get seated on this commercially designated day of love. It was insane. (Mother's Day was even worse!)

I began to dislike V-Day when I became a social worker where I was introduced to my first real office environment. On February 14, our office would look and smell like a flower shop. There were seemingly endless vases of roses and tulips and balloons and teddy bears. Yet it was a sad day for many who didn't receive those deliveries. I found myself getting caught up in it and I remember one year getting mad at my husband for not sending the flowers he got me to the office. How twisted is that? Can you imagine how confused that made him?

A colleague of mine confessed she had flowers sent to herself each year so she wouldn't feel like a loser in front of her co-workers.

V-Day calls for some reframing. What matters is how we treat each other the other 364 days of the year. Find people you love to spend time with. Focus on giving, not getting. Love yourself. And know that being sober and present is the best gift you can give yourself or anyone else you love.

***

Last Monday evening, after hours of planning, two colleagues and I facilitated our first of six pilot classes on trauma. There were 28 students. We experienced a few technical issues—just some of the usual suspects that can happen in virtual teaching land, but nothing we couldn't handle.

And then, my lovely husband decided to reboot the modem in the middle of class because the TV wasn't working, and I was ejected into ether land until he could get the system working again. Even though it lasted only a few minutes, it seemed like HOURS. You might imagine my initial reaction and the look on his face when he realized what he'd done.

I thought the whole Zoom meeting had gone down, which it didn't, thank God, and I was able to rejoin the class.

What does this have to do with sobriety, you may ask?

Everything.

Even though my first reaction to my husband's bonehead move was panic, I immediately took a deep breath and, with a clear head and a rational mind, calmed down and waited to rejoin the class.

I have become that person who doesn't have a complete meltdown when things go wrong. That has EVERYTHING to do with sobriety. Where snowflakes don't turn into snowballs. Hills into mountains. Where I can see things for what they are and make informed decisions. Where a situation that might have turned into a long-lasting argument became something to laugh about. (Although next week, I'm locking Paul in his bedroom until class is over.)

There's a quote in the Big Book of AA that promises this in sobriety:

> "We will intuitively know how to handle situations that used to baffle us." [72]

Yep.

***

Getting sober has made me reflect on people, places and things I haven't thought about in years. This week, I've been thinking about my mother's best friend—Hazel K. She and my mother were inseparable. Our families went on vacation together for years. Those vacations, especially the annual ones to Yosemite National Park, were highlights of my childhood.

Hazel was a strong, tall, red-headed Norwegian woman with the most gigantic, amazing boobs I had ever laid eyes on. I was in awe of them. She always wore a slightly see-through white blouse, and you could see the outline of her bra. She had a special nickname for me: "Miss Piggly Wiggly." (I don't know why giving me a nickname felt so special. It just seemed like such a cool thing.) I often had sleepovers at her house where she would make Krumkake cookies, a Norwegian waffle cookie made of flour, butter, eggs, sugar, and cream baked on a special hot iron. She would sometimes fill them with whipped cream and lingonberry syrup. I think of Hazel whenever I walk into an ice cream shop where cones are baked in-house and the aroma of vanilla is intoxicating.

Everyone else in my life made me feel like I was almost pretty. Almost smart enough. Hazel made me feel like a beautiful and brilliant princess. She had a way of making me feel like I was the only little girl in the world.

And then, at 19, when my nine-month-old daughter died, Hazel came through again. Where others were telling me: "You are so young, you can have more children." "It was God's will." "This was a blessing in a way, because now you can start your life over," and so many other insensitive and inappropriate things that I internalized, Hazel wrote me a letter telling me how she lost her first child and how she managed to live beyond the pain. I was blown away that this had happened to her, too. Her letter came just when I didn't see the point of living without my daughter. I so wish I had kept that letter. Hazel's words gave me the courage to move forward when no one else could.

Sobriety has given me the chance to be a Hazel for others.

Take the time to be a Hazel.

***

Last week I slipped into a behavior that I thought was buried in my pre-sobriety days, and though it may seem like a little thing, it's a rabbit hole I want to avoid going down.

As you know, I teach social work for a local university, and during COVID, there is no staff in the office to print out curricula for virtual instruction. So, I do it myself at home. This makes Paul come unhinged. He starts in on how I'm not getting paid for that; he tells me I need to stand up for myself and demand that I be reimbursed or compensated. "We have a crappy printer, ink is expensive, blah, blah, blah." I admit this happens frequently; curricula are constantly being upgraded, or I'm teaching a brand-new class, but I feel so fortunate just to be able to teach, to be doing what I love during a time when many people are out of work.

So, what did I do?

I started hiding and sneaking it like when I was drinking! I started printing the curricula when he was at work or in the shower. Ridiculous, right? I finally told Paul what I was doing, and he genuinely apologized for making me feel like I had to do that (read as: progress).

"When you know that telling the truth is going to cause the other person to act negatively, it can be tempting to change your story in order to keep things running smoothly and maintain the relationship. We've all done it, and we've seen it work." [73]—Josh King, Psy.D.

This is a reminder that old habits die hard and that the work will be ongoing.

***

I was in a meeting the other day and the speaker was talking about his early exposure to his parents' drinking. It made me think about my parents' monthly pinochle club with about ten other couples, including two sets of maternal aunts and uncles. When it came time for my parents to host, I remember what a big deal these card game socials were in our house.

My parents would go all out setting up the card tables, folding chairs, matching tablecloths, and crystal cut ashtrays. We spent hours preparing appetizers and snacks, my parents' version of modern-day charcuterie. There were bowls of chips, chocolate bridge mix, pastel mints, Chex Mix, Spanish peanuts mixed with candy corn (yuk), trays of little sandwiches, veggie trays, and, of course, a bar fully stocked with all things alcohol, mixers, and garnishes.

My cousin and I loved the covered card tables; they made for great forts until we were discovered and banished to another room after the card games commenced. We were expected to help clean up in the morning. It was gross. The entire house would smell like one giant, disgusting ashtray. There would be spilled and half-filled cocktail glasses, food stains on the tablecloths, and stale potato chips ground into the carpet. To this day, I cannot eat candy corn.

I remember sneaking a drink of my dad's gin and tonic, spitting it out, and wondering why anyone would purposefully put in their body something that had the taste of gasoline. I vowed never again to let alcohol pass my lips.

I can't help but think how all of this influenced my relationship with alcohol and, in turn, my adult children's relationship with it as well. I know that they have few social events that don't include alcohol. It's so acceptable for their age group.

And yet, I don't advocate that everyone should stop drinking. · Lots of my friends and family are normal drinkers. However, I do know that sobriety is trending, and it feels so good to be part of that movement. Alcohol-free bars are popping up all over the world. I love that I can show my grandkids another way.

***

I used to be one of those people who could fall off Mt. Everest, get up and say, "Don't worry about me. I'm okay. Nothing to see here." I was living behind a mask, always trying to keep other people from feeling uncomfortable.

I was good (or so I thought) at masking my pain.

My psychiatrist was the first person ever to call me on it. I remember telling her about losing my daughter. And about how my dad and mom died within 18 months of my losing the baby. After telling her this, I immediately followed with: "But I wouldn't be here if all that didn't happen to me. I wouldn't have the life I have now." (Mind you, this was all before I came clean with the fact that I had an alcohol problem.) She made me stop and realize that I never grieved over any of it. My brother's marriage ended because of the accident; it fractured our family for years, and I just felt I couldn't add to everyone else's pain. So, I buried mine and said, "I'm okay."

As I continued to place more and more unaddressed events into my traumatic backpack, my feelings became too heavy and began leaking out in maladaptive and self-destructive ways. Drinking wine was the biggest one. And then I almost lost everything. Saying

"I'm okay" kept me in the dark for so many years. Being honest and sober allowed for the genuine work to happen. And then the light came in.

***

I have had several opportunities to tell my sobriety story in a variety of settings. And, of course, the self-doubt of imposter syndrome began to creep in. Why would anyone want to hear what I have to say? I can feel like this when I get in front of a classroom to teach, present at a conference, or write. This was even more true when I was drinking. According to Dr. Michael Friedman in Pyschology Today:

> "Imposter syndrome refers to the persistent feeling of doubt that our achievements are justified and reflect our talent, skills, and efforts. We can feel that we are frauds and that our success is somehow not earned. Unfortunately, we are susceptible to imposter syndrome in any and all areas of our lives." [74]

Even when we are alcohol free.

In the work I have done to get and stay sober, I acknowledge that imposter syndrome probably affects everyone at one time or another. When it happens to me now, I consciously breathe and dismiss it from my mind. "Fear" is another word for imposter syndrome. I have learned to use fear as a motivator to keep practicing, preparing, and performing what I believe to be my purpose of writing, teaching, and connecting.

And …

In theory, our purpose is never really completed, right? If I pause for a moment, I know I didn't get to where I am right now through dumb luck. I get to work on my sobriety every day. I know this work will never be done. I am not perfect; perfection is a false construct that only brings on the feeling of being less than. In his book, Healing the Shame That Binds You, John Bradshaw writes:

"Perfection denies healthy shame. It does so by assuming we can be perfect. Such an assumption denies our human finitude because it denies the fact that we are essentially limited. Perfectionism denies that we will often make mistakes and it's natural to make mistakes." [75]

There is not blueprint for being human. There is a certain satisfaction and peace in that for me because life-long learning provides for an existence free from boredom.

***

How many of us have or had young children and wish they would hurry and grow up? Parenting, especially parenting of young children, is really hard work. And then one day we wake up like I did, and our children are suddenly adults, and we wonder where the hell the time went. It's like they grew up overnight. We look back and wish for a do-over.

Whatever age our children, we need to marvel at them NOW.

Sobriety is like that, too.

We need to slow down. One day at a time as they say, right?

If we are in early sobriety, we can get hung up on the outcome rather than the day-to-day challenges and successes.

"Cure your destination disease. Live mostly for today, less for tomorrow, and almost never about yesterday. How? You might have to repeatedly remind yourself that yesterday is gone forever, yet we perpetually have to deal with now, so why not live it? And what if tomorrow never occurs? There is a difference between working towards the future, which is inherently enjoyable in the light of hope, and living in an unrealistic future that remains perpetually unknowable. If tomorrow never comes, would you be satisfied with the way today ended? It is not how you start in life or how you finish. The true joy of life is in the trip, so enjoy the ride!" [76] —Steve Gilliland

Are you having a bad day? Life picks on everyone—we don't need to take it personally.

Remember that AA saying? Your worst day sober is better than your best day drunk.

Just. Don't. Drink. Today.

Chapter 7

In Conclusion …

"It's hard to believe I am the same person.
Oh wait, I'm not." – Peggi Cooney

I have literally put myself and my sobriety journey out there for everyone to see by posting, by going public on Instagram, and by starting my own Facebook page and newsletter. I am putting the finishing touches on this book—one I never knew I would write.

Who knew
I would be thriving as I enter my third year of sobriety,
surrender every day,
create an ever-growing Facebook and Instagram community
full of people who are supporting each other to get and stay
sober,
have my work published in magazines,
write this book.

Who knew
I would be comfortable telling the whole world about my
sobriety journey,
be present,

develop sustainable, healthy coping mechanisms like breathing, mindfulness and journaling, be this quiet on the inside (thank you, Jill Q.),
connect with other humans in a way I never thought possible.

Who knew
I would feel comfortable in my own skin,
be grateful,
value wholeness over happiness,
make my family proud,
love myself sober.

Many people who have followed my story have approached me and said, "I want what you have. I want to be successful at living an alcohol-free life. What should I do?"

Here are a few of my thoughts …

I no longer hope for a better life because I have discovered that hope is not some intangible thing that may or may not happen in the future. In sobriety, hope has become a verb. Something I DO. Make happen. On a daily basis.

My future will always thank me for not drinking today. I chose to change my story. At first, I changed for my family; in the end, I changed my life for me.

Accept that change is uncomfortable. Welcome it. Don't push it away. Work through it. Learning something new requires that we get uncomfortable. You will be okay. You will survive.

Getting sober can be boring at first. And then it isn't. And then it really isn't.

Tell on yourself. The more people who know about what you are doing, the better chances you have at getting and staying sober. Secrets fuel addiction. Shame and guilt can be powerful motivators to pick up that drink again. (Be sure to completely confide in at least one or two people who know everything, in case you go quiet.)

Discover the underlying reasons you drink. Dig deep. There are no Cliff Notes, no magic bullets for sobriety. Everything gets easier when you do the work. This can happen through your own customized combination of working a recovery program, therapy, exercise, self-discipline, and connection. There are so many amazing programs to choose from, you can't help but find ones that will fit you. Life is just better sober.

- Don't be afraid to reach out to someone who resonates with you.
- Listen to people who are where you want to be.
- Surround yourself with sober humans and sober allies.
- Letting go of what was can be painful, but never forget how bad it was.
- Close the trap door. Shut it tight. Lock it. Don't give yourself an out.
- Stop romancing the wine glass.
- Volunteer. We learn how important it is to be of service in sobriety.
- No matter where you are on the alcohol train, you will certainly learn something about yourself when you look at your relationship with it.

Sobriety isn't the goal. Peace, success, self-love, family, stability, spirituality, happiness, and helping others are the goals. Sobriety is the vehicle by which you can achieve these goals or any others you have set for yourself.

Let fear be your ally. Fear is a natural response to change, but I had been letting it lead me, instead of me leading it, for years. I had to take that leap of faith and listen to that voice that had been telling me that if I put in the work, my fear could become my internal guide to the life I wanted and the one my children and grandchildren deserve.

I remind myself that I had used fear to my advantage before. I remember standing in front of my first class of social workers looking and presenting much like a deer in a headlight. I pushed through that fear until I fell in love with teaching.

Fear has become not only my ally; it has become my protector. I am predictable and reliable and present. I am that person who has fallen in love with sobriety. I am that woman who has fallen in love with herself. I still get sad. I get hurt. I hurt other people. I screw things up. I also laugh—full-blown body laughter. This is what being a whole human is all about.

I am no longer addicted to wine. I am no longer 27 versions of myself. And when we are living as who we really are, when we find our dharma, our truth, we naturally become of service to the world.

And, as my very important person Judy says: "This is not about perfection. Do what you can. And if you can't, wake up the next day, straighten out your crown, and keep going. We in the recovery community are always cheering you on. No story you can share will surprise any of us. We've been there! We are you! Okay, I'm stepping off my soapbox. Carry on and get EXTREMELY PSYCHED for a positive change in your beautiful life."

I often walk with Susan on the Sacramento State campus. When we first started walking there, she said we were going to warm up by climbing what looked to me to be an impossible set of stairs to conquer. I said, "No way!" The stairs seemed so daunting at first, but then, with practice, I made it to the top. It became easier with each climb. Just like getting sober. And the view from both is stunning.

What do you want your story to be?

Chapter Eight

After
(21 months)

"There's no real ending,
it's just the place where you stop the story."
—*Frank Herbert*

Aloha. Tomorrow morning, I am leaving on a jet plane to Hawaii, with Paul, Lindsay, Jason, Teagan, Rylan, Jaxson and Sawyer. When we get to Honolulu, there will be no worries about where I can buy wine as soon as we get off the plane. No worries about where I'm going to hide the bottles. There will be no alcohol-fueled incidents that will make Lindsay regret she invited me or make Jason and my grandchildren feel uncomfortable. Paul and I won't get into any arguments because of my drinking. I won't misplace my wallet or lose my driver's license. There will be no hangovers. Only priceless family memories, walks on the beach, swimming, dinners, sunsets, and sunrises. There will be hours of "Hey, Grandma, watch me!" And a family picture with matching Hawaiian outfits that will make a stunning Christmas card for 2021.

***

We arrived at the Sacramento Airport to begin our family Hawaii trip. I saw Lindsay and her family walking up to the gate. I semi-ran to give who I thought was my grandson Jaxson a ginormous hug, practically tackling him to the ground. The thing is, it wasn't Jaxson; it was another little boy. (In my defense, the masks can make it difficult to distinguish your grandson from others.) Lindsay was horrified. Thank God, the kid and his parents thought it was rather humorous.

Haha! At least I wasn't drinking.

We had the best five days at the Aulani Disney. No drama. Only memories. And then Paul and I were off to Maui. There were no rental cars because of COVID. I took a chance and called a sober sister, Ann, who lives in Maui and asked her if she knew anyone who might rent us their car. Well, SHE did. Not only did she rent us her car; she picked us up at the airport with leis and a cooler filled with cold drinks and snacks. We had never met in person before. We are having lunch on Tuesday. The friendships in recovery are real and the best. Ann made our vacation.

And because we didn't think we would have a car, we pre-ordered grocery delivery service and when we arrived at our hotel, our cupboards and refrigerator were stocked with almost everything we needed for the week. We didn't need to stop at Safeway on the way to Napili, where in the past, Paul and I would be bitching at each other because we were tired and couldn't decide what to buy. It was all there waiting for us. It was magical.

So, here we are, having the best second half of our vacation. Paul has discovered he likes my Heineken 00, and I'm enjoying my POG (Pineapple Orange Guava) juice with club soda. Life under the Maui sun is good.

***

We have been home for two days from our Hawaii vacay. Back to reality. Other than the nightmare that traveling with COVID was (I never want to hear the words "QR code" again), this trip to Hawaii was our best so far. Without alcohol. Who ever would have thought that a vacation could be fun without my old BFF?

I really enjoyed the first week, being with Lindsay and her family in the new and improved Peggi way.

Over the last decade, I had fallen into a pattern of doing whatever it took to make Lindsay happy, no matter what sacrifice it was to me. (Sadly, I think the only thing she really wanted was to have a sober mother.) I'm not sure why and how we began this dance. It's like our roles were reversed and she was the parent, criticizing and scolding me as if I were the child. Of course, my drinking had a lot to do with it.

During this trip, I was able to tell her what I needed. On the first night, Paul and I told Lindsay we wanted to get an early dinner on our own because we were exhausted and wanted to get to bed early. Pre-sobriety, I would have waited around for her to decide what she wanted to do.

> "When we feel responsible for other people's feelings, we believe we have to adapt and modify our own behavior, so others are happy and find us acceptable." [77] —Laura McKowen

We had such a nice balance of spending time together with the grandkids (some meals together, swimming, a luau, and babysitting on the last night so that Lindsay and Jason could have an evening to themselves). There were other times when Paul and I spent our own time together, going on walks and reading. It was a perfect balance of together and alone time. There was no drama, no resentments, and a good time was had by all. And I know it may sound like "well, duh," but I felt like my daughter showed more respect for me and appreciated me more. Life just keeps getting better on this side of alcohol.

BTW, so much for those matching Hawaiian outfits for the ultimate Ohana Christmas card. Rylan wouldn't wear hers because it made her skin itchy; Jaxson's shirt was too big and hung down to his knees; Lindsay said she looked like she was wearing a muumuu. (Boy, did that word trigger memories of my mother's embarrassing choice of daily attire.) That left only me, Teagan, and Sawyer with our island apparel. Best intentions, right? And did I mention we had to keep our masks on while posing with Moana and Maui?

***

Sobriety is trending and I am so flipping proud to be part of it. More women (and men) are waking up and saying to themselves, "I don't want to live like this anymore." Parents are asking, "What have I been teaching my son or daughter?" More and more people are rejecting the notion of these popular messages: "Mommy's wine has become pop culture." "Wine is quick. It's easy. Expected." "Life is hard. Wine helps." "Alcohol is self-care. Wine is the antidote for the stresses of motherhood."

In addition to teaching, I have found my place in the recovery community. My Facebook page, This Side of Alcohol, has become a community where people from all over the world come together to support sobriety and the sober curious. I cannot tell you the joy I feel when I see someone post that they need help and immediately there are dozens of supporting messages. I facilitate a weekly recovery support group in the Northern California area; I am a guest host for the Facebook live casts for Getting BAC2zero; and I'm developing a sobriety tool that will help to discover and map the underlying reasons humans turn to alcohol and outline the customized steps to get and stay AF. There are so many ways to get sober these days. I just know my mom is looking down with envy, pride, and awe.

Epilogue

(23 months)

"Find a house where the truth is told."
—Laura McKowen

Whhat happens when your partner reads your memoir for the first time?

I am facing my final hurdle before this book is sent to the publisher: letting my husband read my book. Paul has never read any of the articles I have published. He knows I've written them, but he has never asked to see them. He will be going up to our cabin this week specifically to read my book.

I admit I'm nervous.

I wonder what his take will be on how I've written about us. About our family. Will he understand the addiction behind the thousands of lies I told about my drinking? He says he already knows all about the lies, but does he? Will he understand my feelings as a stepmother? He says he will, but people do judge, even when they say they won't.

During the writing of This Side of Alcohol, I have had constant internal debates of what I could or couldn't say, should or shouldn't reveal, about myself and my family. In my heart, I truly feel that I have been fair to them, to the story, to myself.

Paul and I have agreed on some guidelines, one of them being that he will read the book all the way through before talking about it with me. My book starts out raw and angry and ends up honoring him for choosing to understand addiction over leaving. Will he be able to honor that agreement?

My friend Alice suggested I add that he agrees to read it with an open heart more than an open mind. Check.

We have agreed to discuss any changes he thinks should be made, with me having the final say about whether something stays or goes.

It's no coincidence that yesterday I read the final pages of Mary Karr's brilliant memoir *Lit*.

> "For over two years, Mother hounds me to let her read pages I'm scribbling about the worst patch of our family history ... But I know reading it could hurt them, since writing it often wrings me out like a string mop." [78]

It's comforting, somehow, that I have all of you alongside. My friend Liz wrote: "When Peggi said the last step in writing her book was to let her husband read it, my heart skipped a beat. I understand those words…There are so many layers to shame but putting it out there, trusting that God has a plan to heal you more, is complete surrender."

I have high hopes that coming clean, having no more secrets between us, will connect us on a deeper level. Alcohol has kept our relationship at a distance for the last decade.

I will survive this. I have already survived.

***

I was so worried when Paul went up to the cabin to read my manuscript that I made myself sick. At the same time, I felt such relief from finally being able to tell the truth. It was liberating. I was not expecting that the only thing Paul was concerned about was my use of the "f" word throughout myself story. That totally cracked me up. I am so grateful that despite being such a private person, Paul is willing to share intimate details of our marriage and family life in order to support me on my sobriety path.

In Paul's own words …

What did I think of the book?

It was shocking and, at the same time, enlightening.

Your breadth and depth of deceit were a complete surprise. I knew you were drinking, but there was so much I was unaware of. What I saw were the triggering events: holidays, entertaining friends, and family gatherings. Generally, events were measured by occasions spaced out over time, not a day in and day out occurrence. What you said about the wine bottles is a good example; that you had to be mindful and develop a sort of daily "logistics" plan, for their acquisition and disposal. Or the argument you made for screw caps instead of corks, not just as a matter of daily convenience, but a daily necessity in concealment. This is shocking.

Nonetheless, I knew there were many days when you were just a little bit off, just enough to fuel my suspicion you had been drinking, but these were random and didn't involve what you might term as a trigger. Your speech was off, not really slurring, but more of an unnecessary exaggeration. It's hard to describe; others didn't always see it, but I did. You would flop down on the couch, hog conversations, or talk over people. It was irritating to me, but I chalked it up to lack of sleep, or I would try to ignore your behavior so I wouldn't make others uncomfortable. I didn't want to be confrontational in the presence of company.

I mention lack of sleep because I knew that for years you have had a sleep disorder with the most recent diagnosis that the curve in your spine complicated breathing at night [it did], causing you to be constantly exhausted. I didn't realize that your drinking was exacerbating the problem as well.

I considered other explanations for your behavior— your difficult child and young adulthood you so eloquently described in your book. Being a social worker, a first responder in the field, day after day, working with abused children and adults. You were witness to trauma on an almost daily basis in a system that seemed to inflict even more trauma on children, youth, and families.

Then there were events in your workplace that ended up with you being a whistleblower. You ended up so stressed out, your health so fragile, you were put on medical leave for four months.

All these events and circumstances contributed to my concern for you, your mental health, and your eventual drinking problem. My approach became confrontational. I wanted answers.

On those occasions when I asked if you were drinking, you would constantly tell me "no", say you were just tired, or give me something else as an excuse. Or you would admit to drinking and would stop for periods of time, but not until our arguments were full-blown fights that sometimes became physical. You would accuse me of not loving you. You accused me of hurting you. You told me to get out. I would leave. You would beg me to stay. I would forgive you and return. You always blamed me. I was the asshole. Repeat.

It hurts just broaching the subject of blackouts. I hate the word "blackout"; it's too comfortable. It doesn't describe the ugliness of you passing out. To me, the term connotes going to bed and sleeping it off. What I experienced with you ranged from simply falling asleep at a dinner with guests, to finding you passed out on the floor. I realize for you, that this is the source of your ultimate guilt and shame. But you have moved on; your book is your salvation, the product of your hard work and utilizing every tool available. But for me, at the time, the blackouts, and the possibility they would continue became too much to bear and desperation took over. This was the evening of July 12, 2019.

That night in Lake Tahoe, I had had enough. I found myself shouting at Lindsay and Brett to come see their mother lying passed out on the bed and all hell broke out. I was thinking I needed their help, to see the pain I was experiencing, but they didn't understand. They had no idea how bad things had been for me. Brett came after me physically. At that instant, I realized the marriage was over. I was filled with rage and anger. I left. I never wanted to see any of them again.

While we were separated, you asked me to read This Naked Mind and Alcohol Explained. I was skeptical, but I agreed. Eventually, reading these books changed everything for me, but not right away.

Hurt and very discouraged, I confessed to G and L that I had left you and prepared a list of the blackout incidents over the past years. Together, they prepared a list of their own. I didn't actually see their list, nor did they see mine. All in all, the point was made that alcohol was the problem. Naturally, they took my side and wanted to support me in any way they could.

Should I have opened up to them? Maybe not, but in my anger, I did anyway. I should have known that doing so would shut another door. It had happened before, and I know it was like a punch in the stomach to you. But at the time, I wanted to lash out. You caused me all this pain and I wanted you to pay for it. I know that making amends between you and G and L is going to be very difficult. Whether or not my daughters will ever understand the seduction of alcohol is still an open question to this day.

I think most people understand the dangers of alcohol and are able to control their consumption so that it doesn't have a negative impact on their lives. I may be wrong. Where does control of alcohol end and addiction begin? I know that your relationship with alcohol was not always what it ended up being during the last decade. I know that after reading Annie Grace's and William Porter's books, your addiction to alcohol wasn't your fault. I also know these books saved our marriage.

Peggi, I believe your book will help so many people. You already have.

I know one thing: alcohol is a drug just like cocaine, methamphetamine, and heroin. How can I hold you responsible for your actions under the influence of the most powerful legal and socially acceptable drug in history?

What has your book given me? The realization that no matter how much pain I was feeling, and the lack of understanding I provided, I know your life had become a living hell, a living hell that was not your fault. I hope G and L will come to the same conclusion.

I have become and will remain your biggest fan.

I am so proud of you.

I love you.

Paul

Peggi Cooney
Acknowledgements

"I think new writers are too worried that it has all been said before. sure it has, but not by you."
—Asha Dornfest

There are no words to describe what has happened to my life since Jennifer Kautsch, her dog Franklin, and Sober Sis popped up on my Facebook page on July 12, 2019. How do you express gratitude for someone who showed me the way to save my own life? A leader, a friend, who has been walking beside me since day one. When I started with Sober Sis, there were about a thousand followers on your Facebook page. Today, when I looked, there were 12.3K. Can you say "INFLUENCER"? Without you, Jenn, This Side of Alcohol would not be a thing.

On February 8, 2020, I traveled to San Francisco to meet with a group of Nor Cal Sober Sis women for lunch, followed by a trip to a bookstore to see Laura McKowen, author of We Are the Luckiest. I watched her get up in front of a couple hundred women (I admit, I was star-struck—I had already read WATL three times) to read an excerpt from her book to an audience all connected by a desire to change/understand their relationship with alcohol. That day, Laura's words moved me and many others to tears. I said to myself, "I want that! I want to be in a bookstore, standing in front of people, reading a passage from my own book." Sitting there, I heard a voice answer: "You can do this. You can do this, too."

Here I am.

To all of the people in the unselfish and supportive communities of Sober Sis, The Luckiest Club, AA, Soberish, HOLA Sober, Pandemic Sober Squad, BAC2zero, This Side of Alcohol, and the Nor Cal Zoom Meetings who have encouraged me to put my musings into book form. The list of names to thank would be longer than this book. It's such a cliché, but I really couldn't have done this without you. Y'all know who you are. "Peggi, you really need to turn all of these posts into a book." "You have a beautiful, honest writing style." "Love you, Peggi Cooney. I read two newspapers and your posts every morning." And this: "I didn't pick up that glass of wine tonight after reading your post today."

To my university chair, Susan, and to my directors, Nancy and Alison, who made it safe for me to make public a very serious health issue.

To Judy Matuk, who I accused of "being in my head" after the first of many edits. Thank you for sending those messages like "Okay, I'm going to say something that I don't want you to be mad at me about" and "Don't mess with my changes to the use of the word, 'myriad' (I know I'm right)" and "We will just have to disagree on some of those dangling participles and most of the commas." Your words only served to improve my writing. I was so excited to read your final comment, "Now THIS is a book!!!!"

To Robyn Flemming, my new Aussie friend, author of Skinful: A Memoir of Addiction. I am not sure how the universe brought us together, but I am so glad the stars aligned to make that happen.

To my business coach and dear friend Kaitlyn (Kaitlyn Ash Coaching & Consulting), for designing, developing and maintaining all things social media for This Side of Alcohol. There are really no words. (We do make a great team.)

To Robin Nelson from Leaning Rock Press (Thank you, Judy, once again). Thank you for making my first publishing experience such a painless one. You are a gift.

To Keri Aoki Photography who brought my book cover to life.

To my dear, dear friend, Alice Parvin, who has been my absolute rock, believing I could write this book when every other day I wasn't so sure. Thank God for the Sober Sis retreat that brought you into my life.

To my beta readers: Melinda, Lucy, Jeff, Cathy, Matthew, Jan, Karen, Kezia, Kaitlyn, Valorie, Rosemary, Robyn, Stacy, and Louise. Thank you all for your encouragement, editorial assistance and ongoing support.

To my children and significant others: Matt, Michelle, Lindsay, Jason, and Brett for supporting me in telling my sobriety story out loud.

To my grandchildren: Luke, Kate, David, Lucie, Teagan, Rylan, Faye, Noah, Mia, Alix, Jaxson, and Sawyer. Know that being present and authentic are far greater priorities than the "buzz" that alcohol provides.

To Glenn Ann, Greg, Laura and Pascal: I hope you will remember the good times, too.

To my brothers and sister-in-law's: Jim, Karen, Jerry, Linda, Bob and Monica. For so, so long, we have only had each other.

To Gretchen Stolberg-Vallejo, my first adult best friend. There are no words to describe what it means to have you back in my life. I can't wait to see what the future will bring for us.

To my OG sisters from the August 2019 Sober Sis 21 Day Reset group: Ashley, Beka, Cindy, Colleen, Dolores, Ellen, Jan, Jane, Janet, Joy, Julann, Karen, Kelly, Laura, Lindsay, and Robin. Kelly always said that God handpicked this group of amazing women from all over the country. I believe that to be true.

To those of you who are reading this section and wondering "Where's MY acknowledgement, Peggi?", I can assure you that I am fully aware how you warmly surrounded me with support and helped guide my hand in writing this book. In gratitude, I think it best for me to channel the great Steve Martin when I say that I want to thank each and every one of you: Thank you, Thank you!

And most of all, to the people around the world who are in active addiction. I pray every night that you will find your way back.

About the Author

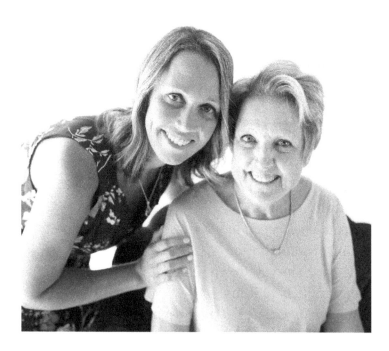

Peggi Cooney is a social work instructor/coach. Peggi has a Master's in Social Work from California State University, Chico, and spent 16 years in Child Welfare and Adult Protective Services as a social worker. Since getting sober, Peggi has become a sobriety advocate and has developed quite a following through Facebook, Instagram, and her website This Side of Alcohol. She facilitates a weekly community support group and is currently working on the development of a recovery program for parents involved in the child welfare system.

Peggi has been married to Paul for 35 years. Together, they have five children and 12 grandchildren. She lives in West Sacramento and Lake Almanor, California. *This Side of Alcohol* is her first book.

www.thissideofalcohol.com
Facebook.com/groups/thissideofalcohol
@thissideofalcohol

Resources I used to get and stay sober.

Apps
Insight Timer (Yoga Nidra with Jennifer Piercy)

Books/Publications

AFTER Magazine
Alcohol Explained: William Porter
Atomic Habits: James Clear
Bird by Bird: Anne Lamott
Blackout: Sarah Hepola
Conversational Intelligence: Judith Glaser
Drink: Ann Dowsett Johnston
Drinking: A Love Story: Carolyn Knapp
Falling Upward: Richard Rohr
Forsyth Woman Magazine: Keela Johnson
Hallelujah Anyway: Anne Lamott
Highlight Reel: Emily Paulson
HOLA Sober Magazine: Susan Christina
Intoxicating Lies: Meg Geiswite
Girl Walks Out of a Bar: Lisa E. Smith
Group: Christine Tate
I Am Just Happy to Be Here: Janelle Hanchett
Journey to the Heart: Melody Beattie
Journey Magazine
Lighter: yung pueblo
Lit: Mary Karr
Look Alive Sis!: Jenn Kautsch
Mocktail Party: Diana Licalzi/Kerry Benson
Mother Hunger: Kelly McDaniel
My Fair Junkie: Amy Dressler
My Unfurling: Lisa May Bennett
Nothing Good Can Come from This: Kristi Coulter
On Writing: Stephen King

Push Off From Here: Laura McKowen
Skinful: A Memoir of Addiction: Robyn Flemming
The History of Love: Nicole Krauss
The Listening Path: Julia Cameron
The Sober Lush: Amanda Eyre Ward and Jardine Libaire
This is How You Heal: Branna Wiest
This Naked Mind: Annie Grace
To Bless the Space Between Us: John O'Donohue
Under Our Roof: Madeleine Dean/Harr Cunnane
We Are the Luckiest: Laura McKowen
What Happened to You?: Bruce D. Perry M.D., Ph.D./Oprah Winfrey
Why Can't I Drink Like Everyone Else?: Rachel Hart
You Are Not Stuck: Becky Vollmer

Drinks (AF)

Athletic Brewing
Better Rhodes; Alcohol free Marketplace
Clausthaler Dry Hopped NA beer
Fever Tree tonics (my favorite is pink grapefruit)
Gruvi IPA NA Beer
Gruvi Prosecco and Bubbly Rose
Heineken 00
Joyus
Lyre
Prima Pave
Raising the Bar
Ritual
Spindrift sparkling water
Spiritless
Spirits Tequila
Topo Chico sparkling mineral water
Twisted Shrub Apple Cider Vinegar Mixer-Elixirs

Podcasts/Lives

BAC2zero/Jeff Graham

Champagne Problems
Rachel Hart
Home Podcast: Holly Whitaker/Laura McKowen
Telling On Ourselves: Lynn, Bre and Vikki
Tell Me Something True: Laura McKowen
The Art of Growth: Joel Hubbard/Jim Zartman
This Naked Mind: Annie Grace
The Unruffled Podcast: Sondra Primeaux/Tammi Salas

Programs
Staci Danford: The Grateful Brain/The Gratitude Boost/Chemical Soup
Annie Grace: This Naked Mind 100 Days of Lasting Change
Joel Hubbard and Jim Hartnell: Art of Growth Enneagram Coaching
Jenn Kautsch: Sober Sis 21 Day Reset
Jenn Kautsch: Alcohol-Free Living Course
Jenn Kautsch: P365
Laura McKowen: We Are the Luckiest: Sobriety in Full Color
Laura McKowen: We Are the Luckiest Academy
Laura McKowen: The Luckiest Club online meetings and community
Michael "Mac" McNamara: Post Traumatic Winning

Products
How Am I Feeling? Conversation Cards (eeBoo)
Icebreaker (Best Self)
The One Thing Core Values Cards (Best Self)
Our Generation Toys (Target)
Our Moments Family Conversation Starters (Our Moments)
Rae Dunn Journals ($7 at TJ Max/Homegoods)
Staedtler Triplus Fineliner Pens
Table Talk Conversation Cards (Manners & Co)

Songs
"Cloudy Day": Tones and I
"Evermore": Taylor Swift
"Every Breaking Wave": U2

"Fee Good": Mukhlis, Jhon
"For Good": Leann Rimes
"Happy": Pharrell Williams
"Happiness": Taylor Swift
"I'm Still Standing": Elton John
"I Love Me": Meghan Trainor
"Me Too": Meghan Trainor
"Rise Up": Andra Day
"One Day at a Time": Joe Walsh; The Eagles
"Speak Now": Leslie Odom Jr.
"We Can Do Hard Things": Tish Melton
"Yes, Yes We Can": The Pointer Sisters
"You Go Down Smooth": Lake Street Dive
"You Make Me Feel Like a Natural Woman": Aretha Franklin

Miscellaneous

Insight Timer App
Ocean Beach Café: San Francisco (Josh the Non-Alcoholic Bartender)
Sans Bar: Austin (Chris Marshall)
The Surrender Novena (Fr. Dolindo Ruotolo)
Zero Proof Experiences - Sober in the City

ENDNOTES

1. Cummins, Talitha, *The Five Best Ways to Talk to Mum About Her Drinking*, (May 10,2017), https://www.llmedium.com>hellosundaymorning.

2. Weller, Rebecca, *The Happier Hour*, Mod by Dom, 2016.

3. Pooley, Clare, *The Sober Diaries*, Hodder & Stoughton, 2019.

4. Grace, Annie, *This Naked Mind*, Avery; 1st edition, 2018.

5. Vale, Jason, Kick the Drink, Crown House Publishing; Reprint edition, 2011.

6. Kautsch, Jenn: https://www.sobersis.com

7. Vidaurri, Tabitha, "Why Drinking Makes Your Anxiety Worse", Tempest, (retrieved September 19, 2021), https://www.jointempest.com>resource-and-anxiety

8. Murray, Mina, Daily Journal: Journaling is Like Whispering to One's Self and Listening at the Same Time, G. Simpson Press, 2021.

9. McKowen, Laura, *We Are the Luckiest: The Surprising Magic of a Sober Life*, New York Library, 2020.

10. IBID McKowen,

11. Whitaker, Holly, Quit Like a Woman, The Dial Press, 2019.

12. McKowen, Laura, (2020) We Are the Luckiest: The Surprising Magic of a Sober Life, New York Library.

13. Koschalk, Katie, *Why Moderation Never Worked,* https://www.kaiekoschalk.com/2019/10/4/why-moderation-never-worked

14. Author unknown.

15. Rocca, Lucy, Glass Half Full, Accent Press, 2015.

16. Gilbert, Alicia, *Sobriety in the Time of Quarantine: Tips for Staying Sober*, Soberish.co, (retrieved September 19, 2021), https://www.soberish.co> sobriety-quarantine

17. Hepola, Sarah, *Blackout: Remembering the Things I Drank to Forget*, Grand Central Publishing, 2015.

18. Asgard, Majid, *Medical Doctor Urges Alcohol Moderation During Pandemic to Maintain a Healthy Immune System"*, *Loyola* Medicine, (April 2, 2020), https://medicine.org.

19. Shonin, E., VanGordon W., & Griffiths, MD, *Can Mindfulness be Addictive?*, DrMarkGriffiths, (October 24, 2016), https://www.drmarkgriffiths.wordpress.com

20. Carroll, Lewis, *Alice's Adventure in Wonderland*, Reader's Library Classics, 2021.

21. Wright, Annie, *How to be a Woman*, GURU Light e-Publish, 2012.

22. Doyle, Glennon, *Untamed*, Random House Publishing, 2020.

23. Clear, James, *Atomic Habits*, Penguin Publishing Group, 2018.

24. McKowen, Laura, *We Are the Luckiest: The Surprising Magic of a Sober Life*, New York Library, 2020.

25. McKay, Hugh, *Wholeness Overhappiness*, https://www.aliveinthefire. com>blog, 2014

26. Robbins, Tony, 2017, https://www.youtube.com/watch?v=nqw0FZdQl-k

27. Francis of Assisi Quotes, BrainyQuote.com, BrainyMedia, https://www/brainyquote.com/quotes/francis_of_assisi_121465, 2021.

28. McKowen, Laura, *We are the Luckiest: The Surprising Magic of a Sober Life*, New World Library, 2020.

29. Elizabeth, Jenn, *Shape of a Woman*, Maddix Publishing, 2019.

30. Lamott, Anne, *Anne Lamott: I Love Her*, Pip Wilson, *https://www.pipwilson>2015-7-anne-lamott-I-love-you, 2015.*

31. Rohr, Richard, *Transforming Pain,* (October 17, 2018), https://cac. org>transforming-pain-2018-10-17

32. Liv's Recovery Kitchen, *4 Powerful Stories of Transformation*, blog,

https://www.livsrecoverykitchen.com/articles>4-powerful-stories-of-transformation

33. Gilbert, Alicia, *The Myth of Moderation*, https://www.aliciamars.medium.com, 2016.

34. Bacharach, Burt & David, Hal, *What the World Needs Now Is Love*, as performed by Jackie DeShannon, https://www/lyrics.com/lyric /6109775/Jackie+DeShannon/What+the+World+Needs+Now+Is+love

35. Whitaker, Holly, *Quit Like A Woman*, The Dial Press, 2019.

36. Boehm, Traver, *One Day Stronger*, https://www.traverboehm.com>ods-starts-here., 2019.

37. McClaren, Karla, *The Language of Emotions: What Your Feelings are Trying to Tell You*, Sounds True, 2010.

38. Johnston, Ann Dowsett, Drink, Harper Wave; 1st edition, 2013.

39. AAWS, Big Book of AA, Alcoholics Anonymous World Services, 4th edition, 2001.

40. McKowen, Laura, *We Are the Luckiest: The Surprising Magic of a Sober Life*, New York Library, 2020.

41. Doyle, Glennon, Untamed, Random House Publishing, 2020.

42. Clear, James, Atomic Habits, Penguin Publishing Group, 2018.

43. McKowen, Laura, *We Are the Luckiest: The Surprising Magic of a Sober Life*, New York Library, 2020.

44. Glaser, Judith, Conversational Intelligence, Routledge, 1st edition, 2016.

45. ibid, Glaser

46. Peters, Megan, *5 Tips to Keep Your Relationship Together While Getting Sober*, Tempest, https://www.thetemper.com, 2018

47. Glaser, Judith, *Conversational Intelligence*, Routledge; 1st edition, 2016.

48. Benson, Carly, *Sobriety Requires Surrender, Miracles Are Brewing*,

(October 22, 2014), https://www.miraclesarebrewing.com

49. Seuss, Dr., *Oh, the Places You'll Go!*, New York Random House,1990.

50. Hanchett, Janelle, *I'm Just Happy to be Here,* Hanchett Books, 2008.

51. McKowen, Laura, *We Are the Luckiest: The Surprising Magic of a Sober Life*, New York Library, 2020.

52. Clear, James, *Atomic Habits*, Penguin Publishing Group, 2018.

53. Ibid, Clear, James.

54 Henneke, *Being vs Doing: The Peculiar Art of Getting Unstuck*, (retrieved September 20, 2021), https://www.enchantingmarketing.com

55. Campbell, J., Flowers, B.S., & Moyes, B., The Power of the Myth, Doubleday, 1988.

56. Wyse, Lois, (retrieved September 20, 2021), https://www.goodread.com

57. Brault, Robert, *Round Up the Usual Subjects*, Createspace, 2014.

58. Knapp, Caroline, *Drinking: A Love Story,* Dial Press Trade Paperback, 1997.

59. Rietz, Katie, *Does Your Partner Resent Your Recovery?,* The Fix, (August 31, 2018), https://www.thefix.com

60. Ashton, Jackie, *10 Simple Things to Make You Happier at Home,* Apartment Therapy, https://www.apartmenttherapy.com

61. My Childhood Punishments Meme, (September 19, 2016), https://www.dansversion.com/2016/9/19/my-childhood-punishments-have-become-my-adult-goals/

62. Ward, Amanda and Jardine Libaire, *The Sober Lush.* TarcherPerigee, 2020.

63. Caddell, Jenev, *How to Express Your Needs in a Relationship*, (retrieved September 19, 2021), https://mybestrelationship.com

64. Rogers, Megan, *Saying No to a Party Social Life in Early Sobriety*, (May 24, 2019), https://www.megan-rogers.com

65. Author unknown.

66. Gilbert, Alicia, *The Case for Adopting a Strong Morning Routine,* Soberish, https://www.soberish.com>morning-routine-sobriety, 2021.

67. Vidaurri, Tabitha, *Why Drinking Makes Your Anxiety Worse,* https://www.jontempest.com>resourse-and-anxiety, 2021.

68. Eisold, Ken, *Good Anxiety – And Bad,* Psychology Today, (February 21, 2020), https://www.psychologytoday>hidden-motives

69. The Joy Blog, *How to Actually Take Things One Day at a Time,* http://www.thejoyblog.net>how-to-actually-take-things-one-day-at-a-time, 2015.

70. Quindlen, Anna, (2000), *Anna Quindlen's Commencement Address at Villanova,"* http://www.cs.oswego.edu.>wender-quindlen, 2000.

71. Tate, Christie, *Group,* Avid Reader Press / Simon & Schuster, 2020.

72. AAWS, *Big Book of AA, Alcoholics Anonymous World Services;* 4th edition, 2001.

73. King, Josh, *How to Talk When You Think They Are Lying,* Motivational Change, (August 14, 2017), https://www.motivationalchange.com>how-to-talk-when-you-think-they-are-lying

74. Friedman, Michael, Ph.D., *How to Rock Your Imposter Syndrome,* Psychology Today, https://www/psychologytoday.com

75. Bradshaw, John, *Healing the Shame That Binds You,* Health Communications, Inc., Expanded and updated edition, 2005.

76. Gilliland, Steve, *Understanding the Destination Disease,* https://www.stevegilliland.com>understanding-the-destination-disease

77. McKowen, Laura, *We Are the Luckiest: The Surprising Magic of a Sober Life,* New York Library, 2020.

78. Karr, Mary, *Lit,* Harper Perennial, 2010.